The Organization of
Soviet Medical Care

MICHAEL RYAN

The Organization of Soviet Medical Care

Special edition published by
Professional Seminar Consultants, Inc.

© Michael Ryan 1978

First published in 1978 by Basil Blackwell & Mott Ltd.,
Oxford and Martin Robertson & Co. Ltd., London

British Library Cataloguing in Publication Data

Ryan, Michael
  The organization of Soviet medical care. –
  (Aspects of social policy).
  1. Health services administration – Russia
  I. Title   II. Series
  361.1′0947   RA395.R9

  ISBN 0–631–18140–7

Contents

About *Professional Seminar Consultants, Inc.*

Professional Seminar Consultants, Inc. (PSC) was established in 1967. The organization was formed to develop a base for international educational programs involving American physicians. Tens of thousands of health professionals have been involved in more than 1,000 programs since that beginning. During 1978, preliminary plans were formulated to extend and formalize the educational experience for all participants. Advance preparation of a syllabus, translation of papers into foreign languages, and the analysis of program evaluations, developed systematically. The Office of Continuing Professional Education (OCPE) was established in 1979.

OCPE/PSC has several educational functions. The main effort is directed toward international clinical study programs. OCPE is dedicated to excellence in educational planning of continuing professional programs in different cultural settings which focus on the common concern of improved patient care.

OCPE/PSC is involved in a foreign educator program bringing outstanding clinicians, from different countries around the world, to the United States.

OCPE/PSC is involved in the publication of selected educational materials.

OCPE/PSC, as the international connection, is involved in linking educational organizations, professional organizations and specialty societies with their counterparts in other countries around the world. This effort is designed to extend our interest in comparative research between health care systems in different cultural settings.

OCPE/PSC is interested in developing a traineeship program allowing extended individual study in a foreign setting.

OCPE/PSC wants to extend research in continuing professional education.

OCPE is recognized as an educational organization and accredited for continuing medical education by the American Medical Association. The total program in continuing nursing education has been approved by the Western Regional Accrediting Committee, American Nurses' Association. The American Psychological Association has accredited this organization for professional programs involving psychologists. Specific programs have been reviewed and accredited by various organizations in the health professions having continuing education requirements for their specialty membership. OCPE has initiated a request for national review toward accreditation in continuing pharmaceutical education and continuing dental education.

□

Preface

When our Clinical Study Program to the Soviet Union began in 1968, Professional Seminar Consultants, Inc. (PSC) made a commitment to develop the most effective educational experience possible. International study tours provide a stimulating challenge, offering exciting and rewarding experiences. Even routine events, when seen in new surroundings, have a quickening effect. Through an innovative and stimulating format, we have continually improved and extended our resources for this professional education program.

PSC is dedicated to excellence in planning and conducting continuing education programs in different cultural settings, programs which focus on the common international concern of effective patient care. Several years ago I decided the theme for PSC would be *"Liaison for International Professional Education."* The publication of this book is a concrete example of our continuing effort to develop this international bond between the health professionals of different cultures.

Marvin E. Weisberg,
President
Professional Seminar Consultants, Inc.

Foreword

Health care professionals worldwide share a vital concern for the best available health care system and improved patient care. The impact of different cultures, health care systems, and educational approaches will influence your learning experience. Basic problems of survival and balance in this world link peoples of different nations and cultures. Through comparative study in this international connection, we hope the developments in our various national systems of health care will be shared in a positive way which influences patient care. There is no single best system which can apply to all countries because of the complex historical, geographical, socioeconomic, and cultural differences which comprise our family of man.

It is hoped you will benefit from this unique educational opportunity and approach this Study with an attitude of inquiry. In order to understand advances and various approaches to health care within a specialty area, the total health care system requires your attention. A fuller understanding of the comparative aspects of the American and Soviet health care systems will enable you to define complex issues to which there are no quick answers and oblige you to question issues about the health care system. Health care, as a right and responsibility of government, is written into the constitution of the Soviet Union. The Soviet system is a centrally controlled program placing major emphasis on prevention. In contrast, the American health care system has no comparable governmental declaration, and though under national economic forcing factors, exists as a pluralistic system with heavy emphasis on the diagnosis and treatment of disease.

Michael Ryan is a sociologist from the United Kingdom. In preparation for your Study in the Soviet Union, his text has been selected as one of the elements allowing an understanding of a different cultural setting. Ryan's study is based on direct observation, extensive reading of Soviet literature, and his perspective as a social scientist placing the health service in the context of a total societal system.

This text is an important part of your preparation and we hope you will use the material and the other advance study documents to the fullest advantage, working independently and at your own pace. The time you take to prepare will help you define your needs as an entry to the Clinical Study. We think your learning experience may have an impact on subsequent work with your patients upon return to your professional setting.

On behalf of the professional staff involved in educational planning for this Study, let me wish you an outstanding experience.

John R. Graham, MD, CM, FRCP(C)
Office of Continuing Professional Education
Professional Seminar Consultants, Inc.

CHAPTER 1

The Politico-administrative Context

It is appropriate to begin by emphasizing the significance which attaches to governmental responsibility for the provision of health protection. Soviet textbooks give it considerable prominence, as does the legal code under which the service is currently supplied. This legislation in fact opens with the words: 'Protection of the people's health is one of the most important tasks of the Soviet state'.[1]

As might easily be inferred, state responsibility in this sphere is portrayed as manifesting the attention that a socialist society pays to the material well-being and living conditions of its citizens. The legislation mentioned above, which was adopted in 1969, contains a statement to the effect that the Soviet system of health protection represents one of the greatest achievements of socialism. Similarly the 1961 Programme of the Communist Party of the Soviet Union asserts: 'The socialist state is the only state which undertakes to protect and continuously improve the health of the whole population'.[2]

One of the objections to such doctrinal assertions is that they serve to obscure the fact that public agencies of various kinds played a major role in the delivery of medical care before the Revolution of October 1917. It is worth recording that administratively separate services were provided for limited sections of the population by a number of central government departments including those responsible for internal affairs, trade and industry, education, the armed forces and agriculture. Also active in this sphere were the Boards of Social Welfare, Municipalities and, in European parts of the Empire, Councils of Provinces and Counties.

Of the various public services, apparently only those provided by

5

Provincial and County Councils (the *zemstva*) have been singled out for anything like detailed historical analysis by Soviet scholars. Viewed in an ideological light, this selectivity is predictable. The *zemstva* local government agencies, established under a law passed in 1864, were not the legal agents of the Tsarist central government and their services mainly benefited an 'oppressed class'—the peasants. Moreover, the *zemstva* doctors can easily be represented as exceptionally idealistic by virtue of the discomforts they endured to improve health conditions in backward rural areas. Whether on account of their experiences or prior commitment (or both), many of these individuals held advanced views on social and political questions. A number of specifically Bolshevik doctors worked for the *zemstva*; they included N. A. Semashko who later became the first People's Commissar of Health Protection and Z. P. Solovev, his deputy.

Under the *zemstva* a fairly rapid development occurred in the provision of facilities, with upgrading of existing units and the building of new hospitals and out-patient facilities. It is interesting that an organizational concept which had been pioneered in the Moscow province and subsequently adopted elsewhere still figures prominently in the Soviet system. This is the rural medical sector (*uchastok*), which constitutes the most local of catchment areas for which health care is organized. Another feature common both before and after the Revolution is the reliance on medical auxiliaries, known as feldshers, to undertake diagnosis and prescribe treatment in remoter rural areas which lack fully trained doctors.

The delivery of health care in Tsarist Russia was no more dominated by a powerful and well-organized private sector than it was in Britain before the inception of the National Health Service. That scheme, however, built directly and explicitly on the previously uncoordinated and less than comprehensive public provisions which had developed over a fairly long time-span. It was essentially a product of a broad-based consensus in favour of collectivist reform along evolutionary lines. In a totally different political context, the Soviet health service was brought into existence by revolutionaries as they fought for dominance in the power vacuum which followed the collapse of the anachronistic and incompetent Tsarist government.

The Bolsheviks' struggle to possess Russia necessarily entailed gaining direct control over as many medical personnel and facilities as possible. This is in no way to deny their ideological commitment to public ownership of the means of production and the service industries. It is simply to draw attention to a strategic imperative in specific historical circumstances of social, economic and military chaos.

Although a somewhat arbitrary procedure, the identification of one date to mark the inception of Soviet health protection is obviously useful, and the most appropriate choice lights on 11 July 1918. On that day, the Bolshevik government issued a decree which created a People's Commissariat of Health Protection and vested in it control of all personal and environmental health facilities in the recently designated Russian Soviet Federated Socialist Republic.

By this time, the Civil War was in progress and the Bolshevik government, cut off from grain-producing regions, had to confront the problem of an acute shortage of bread and other basic foodstuffs. Compounding the experience of virtual starvation came the scourge of epidemics. It was no coincidence that on the very day of its creation, the Commissariat of Health Protection was assigned twenty-five million roubles in order to undertake emergency measures against an outbreak of cholera. During the first few months of its existence, the Commissariat gave attention to programmes to counter tuberculosis, venereal diseases and influenza, among other matters.[3] But one of the gravest threats faced by the new regime was the pandemic of typhus. This is referred to in Lenin's well-known and colourful epigram contained in a speech delivered to the Seventh Congress of deputies in 1919. 'Comrades,' he said, 'every attention must be given to this question—either the louse will defeat socialism or socialism will defeat the louse.'

In addition to demands—impossible to meet at all adequately—for control of infectious diseases, an urgent claim on slender medical resources was made by the units of the Red Army. Fighting for control of the country lasted for about three years in one of the most destructive, ferocious and bloody civil wars ever known. By the time that the government's position had become unchallengeable and the USSR was formally established in December 1922, a truly massive discontinuity existed between the old order and the new. The emergent system of health protection, like other features of the Soviet Union's socio-economic structure, had to be organized virtually from scratch following the revolution and as a direct result of it.

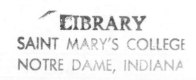

THE MAIN ADMINISTRATIVE STRUCTURE

Given the ideological basis of the Soviet state, it is hardly necessary to make the point that the USSR contains no health care facilities provided by private owners or by religious and philanthropic organizations, such as coexist with the British health service. From the absence of such independent 'competitors' it might be inferred that medical care in the Soviet Union is planned and organized as a single monolithic system capable of securing an optimal distribution of the appropriate buildings, equipment and human resources. That inference appears to be confirmed by grandiloquent statements encountered in textbooks. For example, Maistrakh and Lavrova write: 'All medico-sanitary establishments in the country operate according to a common plan and common methods, are linked together and serve a common objective ...'.[4]

On closer inspection, however, it becomes clear that such assertions deserve to be heavily qualified on various grounds, the most important being that the Soviet Union has not a single organizational framework for the delivery of medical care but several. One of these certainly overshadows all the rest and at this point it is appropriate to devote some attention to describing the administrative context of what can be termed the main health service of the Soviet Union. As might easily be conjectured, responsibility for this system rests not with purpose-designed *ad hoc* public agencies, comparable to those encountered in the British health service, but with the 'organs of state power' which constitute a hierarchical form of local government.

Situated at the apex of the 'organs of state power' is the Supreme Soviet of the USSR, a body comprising two chambers of elected representatives known as deputies. They elect a pro-legislature, the Praesidium, and it is to them and the Praesidium that the Council of Ministers or government is responsible. One member of that Council is the Union Minister of Health.[5] It is an interesting fact that all incumbents of this post have held medical qualifications; at the time of writing the Minister is B. V. Petrovski, an eminent surgeon whose continuing part-time involvement in clinical practice receives publicity in the West. His department, the Ministry of Health of the USSR, is the highest of the 'agencies of state administration' in this field.

Since medical care is a major sector of the USSR's publicly owned and centrally planned economy, wide-ranging powers to control its development are located at Union level. The jurisdiction of the Union, which is specified in detail in the 1969 legislation, relates primarily to the determination of overall priorities, establishment of all-Union plans and the setting of norms to be observed by operational agencies.[6] (Appendix 1 contains a translation of the full text of this law.)

TABLE 1.1   *Population and areas of Union Republics at 1 January 1975*

Union republic	Population (000s)	Area (000 km^2)	Persons per km^2	Population in rural areas(%)
RSFSR	133,741	17,075.4	7.8	33
Ukrainian SSR	48,817	603.7	80.9	41
Belorussian SSR	9,331	207.6	44.9	49
Uzbek SSR	13,689	447.4	30.6	62
Kazakh SSR	14,168	2,717.3	5.2	47
Georgian SSR	4,923	69.7	70.6	50
Azerbaidzhan SSR	5,607	86.6	64.7	49
Lithuanian SSR	3,290	65.2	50.5	44
Moldavian SSR	3,812	33.7	113.1	64
Latvian SSR	2,478	63.7	38.9	35
Kirgiz SSR	3,298	198.5	16.6	62
Tadzhik SSR	3,387	143.1	23.7	62
Armenian SSR	2,785	29.8	93.4	37
Turkmen SSR	2,506	488.1	5.1	51
Estonian SSR	1,429	45.1	31.7	32
USSR	253,261	22,402.2	11.4	40

Source: *Narodnoe Khozyaistvo SSSR v 1974g.*, pp. 16–21.

There can be no doubt that a considerable degree of uniformity in the Soviet health service results from the exercise of power by the Union Ministry of Health in Moscow. But it is striking and highly significant that a senior medical bureaucrat has recorded a view to the effect that greater rather than less uniformity and central control was desirable (at least in certain matters). Writing about the draft of the 1969 legislation, he expressed the hope that it would 'stipulate the need to work out uniform nation-wide guidelines in the management of medical care'. And he continued: 'This relates not only to administrative policy in itself but also to the sphere of the scientific organization of labour and to a number of regulations which in each republic deal in different ways with one and the same problem'.[7]

The republics referred to in the above quotation are the fifteen Soviet socialist republics which together make up the Union. This is not the place to elaborate on the geographical, economic and ethnic heterogeneity of the USSR, but it is desirable to provide some sociographic data about the population and areas of the Union republics. These data, which relate to the beginning of 1975, are presented in Table 1.1, and a list of the republics' capital cities with their population size can be found in Appendix 2.

As can be seen from the table, there is one republic which stands quite apart from the others—the Russian Soviet Federated Socialist Republic (RSFSR) with nearly 134 million people occupying an area of some seventeen million square kilometres. Next in population size comes the Ukraine with nearly forty-nine millions in a territory of 604,000 square kilometres. All the remaining republics contain less than fifteen million people, although the areas they embrace range widely in extent.

Figures for density of population and the proportion of inhabitants ascribed to rural areas have also been included on the grounds that these have a bearing on the organization of medical care facilities and reveal striking variations. Thus in the Turkmen republic there were only 5.1 persons per square kilometre, which contrasts with 113.1 in Moldavia. As much as sixty-two per cent of the population were living in rural areas in the Kirgiz and Tadzhik republics of Central Asia while the lowest figure—for Estonia—stood at thirty-two per cent. Even that can be regarded as high by Western standards and raises questions about the organizational efficiency and productivity of the Soviet Union's agricultural sector.

As at Union level, so in each republic the highest body of state power is the Supreme Soviet: also replicated are the Praesidium, the Council of Ministers, Minister of Health and his Ministry. Under the 1969 legislation, the jurisdiction of a Union republic includes the power 'to establish republican plans for the development of the health service and the implementation of health-improving measures, to direct the health service organs and institutions of a Union republic, to adopt legislative acts in the field of the health service ...'.[8]

Complicating the 'administrative-territorial structure' below Union republic level come the so-called autonomous republics. Each of these has its distinctive ethnic and linguistic character;

they number twenty in all, sixteen of them being located within the RSFSR. Despite the nomenclature, they are to a large extent subordinate to the Union republic in whose territory they are situated. Certainly so far as medical care is concerned, it is entirely proper to locate autonomous republics directly below Union republics on an organization chart. The 1969 legislation specifically states: 'Ministries of Health of Union republics direct the health service through the Ministries of Health of autonomous republics and the health service organs of executive committees of the respective local Soviets of workers' deputies ...'.

The largest of the 'local' administrative-territorial units are the regions (*oblasti*) and the territories (*kraya*). There are 120 of the former and six of the latter. The only but essential difference between a region and a territory is that the latter may include an autonomous region; these amount to a total of eight.[10] Reference should also be made to the ten national areas (*okruga*) which consists of areas inhabited by small ethnic groups in the far north and far east of the USSR. In certain republics, none of these three types of unit are encountered and the line of command proceeds straight down from republic to district (*raion*). As for the towns, the size of their population determines the level of subordination at which they are located. The large towns whose population exceeds 100,000 contain subdivisions for which the term 'district' is also employed.

At these more local levels not all Soviets control their own health department. By 1960 the functions of almost all rural district health departments had been transferred to the district-centre hospital whose chief doctor acquired an additional role as chief medical administrator for the area. It is also the case that health departments have been abolished in certain towns and their work absorbed into one of the large hospitals of the town, with a corresponding alteration in the chief doctor's job description.[11]

At all levels in the main health service except the very highest, health ministries or departments are subject to what is termed 'dual subordination'. Thus although each executive agency is directly answerable to the organ of state power at its own level, it also operates within a framework of regulations laid down by the health department or Ministry which occupies an immediately superior position in the hierarchy. The 'horizontal' subordination is held to afford an effective two-way link between the health service and all other aspects of the socio-economic structure controlled at a given administrative-territorial level. At the same time, 'vertical' subordination permits direction over a whole range of issues which bear directly on the planning and management of medical care.

So far in this brief description no mention has been made of the Communist Party, an omission for which the appropriate analogy is *Hamlet* without the Prince of Denmark. It is essential to note— although Soviet textbooks tend not to—that the hierarchy of governmental agencies is matched at all levels by a hierarchy of Party committees. This institutional point is directly associated with the paramount influence which the Party exercises on so many aspects of daily life in the Soviet Union.

That the Party does indeed play a separate and decisive role in the government of health protection can be illustrated by reference to an incident which occurred in Azerbaidzhan in 1970. The activity of the Health Ministry in that republic had been subject to sharp criticism on various counts: the organization of in-patient treatment was unsatisfactory, especially in the villages; shortcomings existed in the training of health workers and almost all qualitative indices of health care in the republic were lower than the average for the Union. The Azerbaidzhan Central Committee of the Party concluded that their Minister of Health had 'lost the ability to evaluate critically his own activity and the work of his subordinates...'.[12] As a consequence, he was dismissed from his post.

The foregoing account of the structure of the main health service, which was necessary in itself, also has a bearing on the assertion that: 'All medico-sanitary establishments in the country operate according to a common plan and common methods, are linked together and serve common objectives ...'. For it has indicated how multi-tiered and widely dispersed are the responsibilities for planning and management. This point receives further support from the sheer plurality of health ministries and health departments; in July 1971 they amounted to a total of 5,591. As emerges from Table 1.2, and as could be predicted, the majority are at lower levels in the hierarchy: 3,031 for districts,[13] 1,949 for towns and 447 for districts within towns. Although these figures will no longer be precisely correct, the broad impression which they convey remains entirely valid.

Given the size of the country, it is to be expected that local management authorities will be numerous, but fewer would be required,

TABLE 1.2 *Organs of health service administration at 1 July 1971*

Name of organ	Number
Ministry of Health of USSR	1
Ministry of Health of Union republic	15
Ministry of Health of autonomous republic	20
Health Department of autonomous region	8
Health Department of national area	10
Health Department of territory	6
Health Department of region	114
Health Department of district	3,031
Health Department of town	1,949
Health Department of district within town	447
TOTAL	5,591

Source: Kalyu, *Sovremennie problemi upravleniya zdravookhraneniem*, p. 76.

in all probability, if the ideological and political traditions of the USSR permitted the transfer of health service functions from local Soviets to an *ad hoc* purpose-designed organizational structure. Moreover, to pursue conjecture further, such a transfer might reduce the impact of chronic bureaucratic inefficiency in this field. Improving the efficiency of management in the health service, as in other sectors of the economy, has been a high-priority task in recent years and research has indicated the dimensions of the task to be undertaken. Brief mention can be made here of a study undertaken in 1967–71 which used 'tracer methods' to evaluate the effects in local health departments of directives despatched from regional level.[14] The authors found that 'insufficient effectiveness' of orders (*prikazi*) dervied from the following causes:

(a) orders failed to reach their intended destination (50.5% of cases)

(b) material–technical resources were insufficient for their fulfilment (8.2%)

(c) orders lacked concrete instructions (6.8%)

(d) unfavourable consequences (in respect of evaluation of his work) were possible for the person executing the orders (5.8%)

(e) a reduction in functional efficiency was possible (5.8%)

(f) orders repeated directives issued earlier (5.3%)

   (g) different interpretations of orders were made by
      the initiators and the recipients   (4.9%)
   (h) other reasons   (12.7%)

As a further qualification concerning the administrative structure, it must be noted that responsibility for the management of operational units is diffused among authorities at all levels of the hierarchy. Larger hospitals, some out-patient facilities and research institutes are controlled by the region or republic, while some highly specialized institutions are answerable directly to the USSR Ministry of Health. Included among the latter is the well-known and influential N. A. Semashko Institute of Social Hygiene and the Organization of Health Protection. Whatever its origins and justification, this strategy seems unlikely to facilitate consultation and coordination between units which come under separate administrative bodies.

OCCUPATIONAL PROVISION

It is a prominent feature of Soviet health protection that a large volume of medical care is supplied at the place of work. A wide variety of employing agencies make available from their own sources the funds needed to construct polyclinics, hospitals and other units which cater solely or primarily for their workforce. (This arrangement, incidentally, also operates in other fields, including education and housing.) Once constructed, the majority of facilities become elements in the main health service and thus the services provided in them fall under the jurisdiction of the USSR Ministry of Health.

A substantial minority, however, constitute administratively separate schemes which are directed by other ministries, departments and organizations. For ease of identification they can be termed the departmental systems. Although an article of the 1969 legislation states that the USSR Health Ministry exercises a coordinating function over them,[15] in practice they probably enjoy a high degree of autonomy.

The full extent of resources absorbed by the departmental systems remains a matter of conjecture, due to the absence of published data about health care for the armed forces. But a partial account of the commitment of resources can be given for 1970. As is shown in Table 1.3, departmental systems then accounted for 865 in-patient units and it can be calculated that they contained 3.9 per cent of the total recorded number of hospital beds. They also owned 6.7 per cent of premises in which ambulant patients received care and 8.4 per cent of environmental health units. As for staff, who are not included in the table, it emerges from other sources that 12.1 per cent of doctors (including two grades of dentist) were employed in the departmental systems in 1970.[16]

TABLE 1.3 *Health care facilities in 1970*

	In-patient units	Hospital beds	Units for out-patient care	Environmental health stations and departments of district hospitals
Departmental systems	865	104,400	2,347	360
Main health service	25,369	2,558,900	35,013	4,259
TOTAL	26,234	2,663,300	37,360	4,619

Source: *Sovetskoe Zdravookhranenie*, 2, 1972, pp. 85, 88–9.

From one source it appears that the most highly developed departmental systems are those which come under the control of the USSR Ministries of Transport, Defence, Internal Affairs and Civil Aviation and the Committee of State Security (generally known from its initials as the KGB). Polyclinic services for their employees are provided by a number of ministries or governmental organizations including the USSR Ministries of Finance, Foreign Trade, Higher and Intermediate Education, Foreign Affairs, Rural Economy and Aviation Industry. Two polyclinics serve members of the USSR Academy of Sciences and one is situated at GUM, the universal store.[17]

No figures are available to indicate what percentage of facilities in the main health service have been constructed at the expense of mines, factories, industrial plants, agricultural enterprises and the like. However, the contribution is unquestionably substantial and in fact causes disquiet to senior health bureaucrats. As they perceive the problem, dispersed responsibility for planning new facilities can seriously impede the efficient and economic deployment of resources. Thus in 1967 a regional administrator voiced his criticism of the obvious nonsense of building a 480-bed general hospital not far from the 300-bed in-patient unit attached to a motor works in Yaroslavl, and also of the simultaneous erection in Ribinsk of a 500-bed hospital and facilities which included a 250-bed unit at a local factory.[18]

In that year, as it happens, the USSR Minister of Health spelt out a new policy regarding health facilities for workers in productive industry (these facilities consist of polyclinics and other features as well as in-patient accommodation). The essence of this policy was that the 'medico-sanitary units' should be constructed on a larger scale, with not less than 400 beds; industrial enterprises situated in the same locality should combine resources so as to sustain facilities of this size on a joint-user basis. Existing buildings, especially the hospital blocks, should be enlarged at the expense of the enterprise but using standard designs available from the Union Ministry of Health.[19]

Not long afterwards, a comparable attempt was made to foster rationalization of capital investment decisions (with all their logistic implications) in respect of rural health facilities. In July 1968, the Central Committee of the Communist Party of the Soviet Union and the USSR Council of Ministers issued a joint resolution concerning measures to improve health protection and develop medical science. It gave permission for 'the executive committees of Soviets of workers' deputies, with the agreement of enterprises (including state farms) and organizations, situated in rural areas and in the centres of rural districts, and the governing boards of collective farms to *combine the resources* assigned by enterprises (including state farms), collective farms and organizations for the construction of curative and preventive institutions' (my italics).[20]

Whether rural Soviets have used their new powers effectively is not easy to establish but there can be no doubt that in urban areas industrial enterprises have widely disregarded the policy announced by the USSR Minister of Health. For in 1974 B. V. Petrovski found it necessary to criticize the 'tenacious local tendencies' manifest in the provision of small units serving only the workforce of one plant or factory. These he roundly condemned as giving rise to 'squandering of resources, irrational deployment of medical cadres, equipment and apparatus and, in the final analysis, to a sharp decrease in the quality of medical care for the workers'.[21]

It would not be surprising if senior bureaucrats, frustrated by the present limitations on their authority, were actively seeking to restrict the role of enterprises in health care planning. What can be described as the ideal of a tidy administrator was clearly expounded in 1972 by the deputy Health Minister of Estonia.

He started by making the point that during recent years managers of industry and rural enterprises in Estonia had tended to increase the sums assigned for building medical establishments but then went on to question whether the money was being wisely spent. The Minister wrote:

> It is incontestable that health service administrators specifically, and only they, should dispose of the allocations which enterprises make available for the construction of curative establishments in order to allot these resources rationally. The managers of enterprises should understand that departmental tendencies in the health service give rise to splintering which is incompatible with the contemporary level of medicine. The development of specialized care ... is possible only with a maximum concentration of capability and resources.[22]

It is conceivable that the Soviet government, in due course, will enhance the power of health planners *vis-à-vis* managers of enterprises. But the construction of medical facilities at places of work is most unlikely to be abandoned in favour of the strategy pursued in the British health service, whereby all units are open to any person requiring their services, quite irrespective of occupational status. By the same token, the planning process at more local levels will remain to a large extent pluralistic.

CHAPTER 2

Paying for Health Protection

A close relationship exists between the organization of medical services and the methods employed to raise the finance necessary to sustain them. A scheme which is intended to be accessible to all, irrespective of the income of individual patients, must rely very largely on some form of collective prepayment, since payment at time of receipt will have a deterrent effect. In the Soviet Union, as in Britain, the health service is paid for primarily out of taxation raised by the government.

Some Expenditure Data

Official Soviet sources frequently emphasize the fact that expenditure on health protection—and on other social services—has increased substantially from year to year. From the absolute and per capita figures which are cited, the record indeed appears impressive. And there can be no doubt that very considerable improvements of quantitative and qualitative kinds have been made possible by the continuous increase in financial resources.

To draw attention to the annual increases in expenditure on health protection, however, affords only a limited insight into the priority assigned to this form of collective consumption. In the United Kingdom since the mid-1950s it has been common to relate spending on the National Health Service to a measure of national wealth, normally gross national product (GNP). This practice has the obvious advantage of indicating whether a society chooses to spend relatively

18

more on health care as economic growth creates additional prosperity. It is not followed in the Soviet Union and there, as can be calculated, spending on health protection has not risen relative to national wealth over a period of some fifteen years.

This very significant finding emerges from Table 2.1 which is compiled from data contained in the statistical yearbook *Narodnoe Khozyaistvo SSSR*. It will be noted that national income is defined as net material product (NMP). As Michael Kaser points out, this is the measure conventionally employed in Comecon countries and it falls short of GNP 'by the value of services such as administration, the armed forces, health, education, housing and personal service'.[1]

TABLE 2.1   *Expenditure on health protection and physical culture, 1958–1974*

	at current prices				
	1958	1960	1965	1970	1974
Expenditure on health protection and physical culture (milliards of roubles)	5.0	5.7	7.9	11.8	13.7
Net material product (milliards of roubles)	127.7	145.0	193.5	289.9	353.7
Expenditure on health protection and physical culture as a percentage of NMP	3.92	3.93	4.08	4.07	3.87

Sources: *Narodnoe Khozyaistvo SSSR* for 1965, pp. 589 and 783; for 1970, pp. 533 and 732; for 1974, pp. 573 and 758.

NMP data have been published in absolute figures only since 1958, which explains the choice of base-year in the table. The data presented there relate to physical culture in addition to health but the former accounts for relatively small sums and this time-series has the merit of giving expenditure from all major sources—the government budget and a variety of enterprises and organizations. Unfortunately it is unclear whether they include the cost of schemes which were identified as departmental services in Chapter 1.

As the table shows, total expenditure on health and physical culture rose sharply over the period 1958–74, from 5.0 to 13.7 milliard roubles. Expressed as a proportion of net material product, however, the sums allocated to this sector rose marginally from 3.92 per cent in 1958 to 4.08 per cent in 1965 but had fallen back to 3.87 per cent by the end of the period. Due to a variety of methodological difficulties, no precisely comparable figures can be derived for the United Kingdom. However, it would be unduly reticent not to mention that the share of GNP devoted to the National Health Service rose from 3.73 to 5.30 per cent over the same sixteen-year period.[2]

Among the various sources of finance which contribute to the total, only the contributions made by the government budget can be established in precise figures. As might be expected, this constitutes a very sizeable element. In 1974 the sum allocated in the budget to health protection and physical culture was 11.0 milliard roubles, which represented 80.3 per cent of total spending.[3] To assume that the sum in question was expended by health service agencies alone would be reasonable, but there is evidence which appears to imply that other systems receive funds from the government budget to meet the construction costs (but not running costs) of health service units. Thus in 1974 the USSR Minister of Health complained that 'regrettably, a number of industrial ministries (the coal industry, non-ferrous metallurgy, and industrial construction ministries of the USSR) are not fulfilling satisfactorily the plan for constructing curative–prophylactic institutions'.[4]

It is interesting that the cost of constructing or equipping a certain number of health service institutions is met from a type of transfer payment made by employees to the state. This represents the value of work carried out on an unpaid and theoretically voluntary basis on all-Union Communist Saturdays. During the years of the ninth five-year plan (1971–5), this source provided 230 million roubles, which made possible the equipping of various units and the construction of thirty-two children's hospitals with polyclinics attached, three children's polyclinics, eleven maternity homes, thirteen cardiology wards and seventeen general medical wards.[5] No official guidance is given as to whether this specific expenditure is included in the global sums quoted earlier.

In the Soviet Union, in contrast to the United Kingdom, the government does not have to reckon with publicly articulated demands aimed at bidding up the percentage of national wealth devoted to health care. When that has been said, however, it should be added that from time to time the Soviet newspapers report what can be regarded as criticism of the low priority accorded to expenditure on this service. In 1975 an example was provided by an editorial in *Izvestiya*; it stated that 'residents of the settlement of Murmasha in Murmansk region have written to the editor saying that the settlement's population has nearly doubled in recent years but there is still only one polyclinic and this cannot cope with the workload'.[6] During debate on the government budget for 1972 a most revealing complaint was made by one deputy about developments in the Tyumen region of the RSFSR. She said that, in the construction of productive capacity, 'the managers of a number of departments, enterprises and organizations devote insufficient attention to the construction of housing, and social, communal and service facilities'. This was not a new phenomenon, as the speaker revealed when she went on to express anxiety about a situation in which 'the rate of building schools, pre-school institutions, hospitals and other facilities of a social and communal description continues to lag substantially behind the rate of industrial construction'.[7]

Although the regularly published expenditure series relate only to the Union as a whole, it is possible to broaden the discussion by reference to data which are broken down by Union republic. These data come from the government budgets for 1960 and 1970 and exclude the relatively small sums devoted to physical education. It should perhaps be noted that spending which occurs at the various levels in the administrative-territorial structure is taking place within a framework of hierarchical budgets which are subsumed under the Union's consolidated budget.

As they stand, the absolute figures cannot be employed for comparative purposes but when divided by population totals they yield the useful index of per capita spending. Given the combination of a highly centralized form of economic planning and a doctrinal adherence to egalitarianism, it might be supposed that the Soviet Union has achieved a roughly similar level of health care spending per person in each republic. In fact, however, there exists a substantial amount of area inequality.

From Table 2.2 it is evident that in 1960 expenditure ranged from 15.4 roubles per person in the Central Asian republic of Tadzhikistan to 25.3 roubles in Estonia. Ten years later Azerbaidzhan was bottom of the league while Estonia remained at the top and the figures ranged from 27.1 to 41.6 roubles per person. Rather than narrowing, the gap had actually widened by 1970, although of course by then a substantially higher level of spending obtained in all republics.

Almost certainly the gap between the 'haves' and 'have-nots' would have grown less by 1970 had the birth rate and population growth rate been roughly uniform throughout the USSR. As it is, these demographic indicators have varied considerably and the high birth rates

TABLE 2.2   *Government budget expenditure on health protection by Union republic in 1960 and 1970*

Republic	1960		1970	
	Expenditure in millions of roubles	*Per capita expenditure in roubles**	*Expenditure in millions of roubles*	*Per capita expenditure in roubles**
RSFSR	2,408.8	20.0	4,956.3	38.1
Ukrainian SSR	771.5	17.9	1,604.6	34.0
Belorussian SSR	131.7	16.0	290.4	32.3
Uzbek SSR	138.7	16.0	359.8	30.5
Kazakh SSR	175.9	16.9	463.6	35.6
Georgian SSR	75.8	18.1	159.8	34.1
Azerbaidzhan SSR	66.3	16.7	138.7	27.1
Lithuanian SSR	48.2	17.2	113.5	36.3
Moldavian SSR	49.9	16.4	113.0	31.7
Latvian SSR	48.2	22.5	92.7	39.2
Kirgiz SSR	34.7	15.6	94.4	32.2
Tadzhik SSR	32.3	15.4	84.6	29.2
Armenian SSR	31.8	16.8	79.3	31.8
Turkmen SSR	32.2	19.8	68.2	31.6
Estonian SSR	30.9	25.3	56.4	41.6
All-Union budget	700.2	—	532.2	—
TOTAL	4,777.1		9,207.5	

* Sums disbursed under the all-Union budget have been ignored in these calculations.

Source: *Gosudarstvenni Budzhet SSSR i Budzheti Soyuznikh Respublikh 1966–70 gg.*, Finansi, Moskva, 1972, p. 62. Population data were taken from *Narodnoe Khozyaistvo SSSR* for 1960, p. 8; and for 1972, p. 9.

of Soviet Central Asia contrast forcibly with the low rates obtaining in European areas. (The point is one which may be borne in mind when reading comparable accounts of variability in subsequent chapters.) However, while this fact should be recognized, there can be no denying that substantial variation persisted in the figures for per capita spending. In the case of the grosser disparities at least, it seems reasonable to assume that there will also be variation in the quality of medical care available.

To draw an inference about quality from a quantitative indicator may seem to be a highly dubious undertaking. Nevertheless, this particular index can be viewed as a summary measure of a whole set of inputs—doctors and paramedical staff, buildings, equipment and the like—which together play a major part in determining the quality of treatment received by individual patients. There must be a strong presumption that, given the difference in per capita outlays at the start of the 1970s, the health services of Estonia and Latvia were at a different qualitative level from those provided in Azerbaidzhan and Tadzhikistan.

A VARIETY OF INSTITUTIONS

So far the system of health protection has been referred to without attempting to define its content, and this is a suitable point to make good the omission. Only two sub-systems are distinguished in the statistical yearbook, namely: 'curative–prophylactic institutions' and 'sanitary–prophylactic institutions and measures'. The first might be termed personal medical care, although it is essential to note that also included are children's nurseries, children's homes and homes for mothers and children, which are not classified as health service units in the United Kingdom. The second subdivision can be identified as environmental health; in the United Kingdom this is similarly excluded from the National Health Service.

In 1974, the latest year for which data are available, it can be calculated that current spending on personal medical care accounted for the lion's share of total current and capital spending by the government on health protection and physical education. The figure in question was 94.6 per cent, whilst environmental health and physical education absorbed 4.2 and 0.6 per cent of the total. It is clear from Table 2.3 that there remains a further 2.1 per cent of current expenditure in health protection which must be accounted for; this almost certainly relates to non-residential provision for the invalids of the Second World War, bureaux of forensic-medical expertise and various support services.

TABLE 2.3   *Government budget expenditure on health protection
and physical culture in 1974*

Category	Millions of roubles	%
TOTAL	10,966	100
Without capital allocations	10,375	94.6
Out of which:		
curative–prophylactic establishments	9,622	87.7
sanitary–prophylactic establishments and measures	456	4.2
physical culture	60	0.6

Source: *Narodnoe Khozyaistvo SSSR v 1974g.*, p. 759.

Turning now to examine operational units within the main structural divisions, two interconnected features immediately become
obvious. These are the wide range of institutions and the weighting
towards single-specialty rather than multi-purpose functions. This
point emerges from a list which is based on an order issued by the
USSR Ministry of Health in 1949 and updated in 1962. So as to support
the generalization made above and to convey the flavour of Soviet
nomenclature, the list will be quoted in full.

CURATIVE–PROPHYLACTIC INSTITUTIONS

(a) *Hospital institutions*:
   Sector hospital
   District hospital
   District-centre hospital
   Town hospital
   Regional (territorial, republican) hospital
   Hospital for invalids of the Second World War
   Psychiatric hospital
   Tuberculosis hospital
   Infectious diseases hospital
   Specialized hospital [e.g. for convalescence, ophthalmology,
      ENT, psychoneurology]
   Water transport hospital

(b) *Curative–prophylactic institutions of a special type*:
   Leprosy unit

(c) *Dispensaries*:
Anti-tuberculosis
Dermato-venereological
Oncological
Trachoma
Psychoneurological
Physical medicine
Anti-goitre

(d) *Ambulatory–polyclinical institutions*:
Polyclinic
Ambulatory
Stomatological polyclinic
Physiotherapy polyclinic
Health point staffed by doctor
Health point staffed by feldsher
Health point staffed by feldsher-midwife

(e) *Emergency aid and blood transfusion institutions*:
Emergency aid station
Blood transfusion station

(f) *Institutions for maternal and child welfare*:
Maternity home
Collective farm maternity home
Children's nursery
Children's home
Home for mothers and children

(g) *Sanitoria–health resort institutions*:
Sanitorium
Sanitorium–prophylactorium
Health resort polyclinic
Balneological hospital
Mud therapy unit
Sanatorium–young pioneer camp

SANITARY–PROPHYLACTIC INSTITUTIONS

(a) *Sanitary–anti-epidemic institutions*:
Sanitary–epidemiological station
Anti-plague station [probably relates only to animals]
Anti-plague laboratory
Isolation checkpoint [on railways]

(b) *Institutions of sanitary education*:
House of sanitary education

INSTITUTIONS OF FORENSIC–MEDICAL EXPERTISE

Bureau of forensic–medical expertise

PHARMACY INSTITUTIONS

Pharmacy
Pharmacy kiosk
Pharmacy shop
Pharmacy storehouse
Analysis–control laboratory.[8]

Even the foregoing list over-simplifies actuality. Certain types of institution, especially general hospitals and polyclinics, are encountered in duplicate—one for the adult population and the other for children. Moreover, it is possible to identify additional units which are not mentioned in the list possibly because they form an integral part of a larger complex. Examples include consultation centres for maternal and child health, day hospitals attached to psychoneurological establishments and milk kitchens. For budgetary purposes, the system of health protection also embraces clinics situated in higher educational establishments, scientific research institutes, institutes for the advanced training of doctors and stations of the sanitary aviation service.[9]

Owing to the absence of published information, it is impossible to indicate with precision how the health budget is divided as between the many types of institution, let alone as between the services which cater for various population groups and disease categories. The latest breakdown which is at all detailed relates to the republican budgets in 1970; it is presented in Table 2.4. This records current expenditure of 6,366.3 million roubles on what can be identified as the core of the personal health service: hospitals (including their associated out-patient facilities), maternity homes and dispensaries. It can be calculated that operational units located in urban areas and workers' settlements absorbed eighty-three per cent of that figure while rural units received only seventeen per cent. Current expenditure on these core services constituted 73.4 per cent of the total expenditure on health protection under the republican budgets.

It can be seen that the table also records a breakdown of total spending under the eleven main categories which are employed throughout the health service in connection with the standard

TABLE 2.4 Expenditure on health protection by major categories in republican budgets in 1970

| | TOTAL EXPENDITURE | | Current expenditure on hospitals, maternity homes and dispensaries | | | | | |
| | | | Urban and rural areas | | Urban areas and workers' settlements | | Rural areas | |
CATEGORY	Millions of Roubles	%	Millions of Roubles	%	Millions of Roubles	%	Millions of Roubles	%
TOTAL*	8,675.3	100	6,366.3	100	5,284.2	100	1,082.1	100
Out of which:								
Salaries	4,675.6	53.9	3,588.8	56.4	2,992.0	56.6	596.8	55.2
Addition to salaries†	243.2	2.8	198.3	3.1	165.8	3.1	32.5	3.0
Administrative and maintenance expenses	685.7	7.9	568.0	8.9	470.2	8.9	97.8	9.0
Official assignments and journeys on duty	20.9	0.2	14.7	0.2	11.3	0.2	3.4	0.3
Expenditure on food	919.5	10.6	816.3	12.8	663.6	12.6	152.7	14.1
Purchase of drugs and dressings	733.4	8.4	589.0	9.2	488.8	9.2	100.2	9.2
Purchase of equipment and appliances	192.9	2.2	131.3	2.1	109.6	2.1	21.7	2.0
Centralized capital allocations	383.8	4.4	—	—	—	—	—	—
Non-centralized capital allocations	68.6	0.8	—	—	—	—	—	—
Purchase of soft furnishings and uniforms/clothing	232.2	2.7	215.1	3.4	176.1	3.3	39.0	3.6
Repairs to buildings and plant	258.2	3.0	206.7	3.2	171.4	3.2	35.3	3.3

*The total of 8,675.3 million roubles excludes expenditure under the all-Union budget identified in Table 2.2.

†This item appears to cover social security payments to staff.

Source: Popov, Ekonomika i planirovanie zdravookhraneniya, p. 293 (with minor alterations).

budgeting–accounting process. As would be expected in a labour-intensive service industry, salaries account for the lion's share (53.9 per cent), with food (10.6 per cent) and medicines (8.4 per cent) coming a long way behind. In a given institution, budgetary estimates of spending under these and other sub-headings are arrived at by reference to national norms applicable to that size and type of unit. If underspending occurs in one category, as it frequently does, a diversion of resources to another can take place only with the permission of a superordinate agency, an arrangement which has been subject to much criticism in recent years. One textbook claims that this restriction 'infringes upon the rights of a director of a health service institution, delays the timely solution of various questions and frequently leads to the irrational use of allocated finance'.[10]

Health Service Charges

It is an ideological imperative for the Soviet government to emphasize that it makes medical care available to the whole population free of charge at time of use. The high cost of treatment which has to be borne directly by patients elsewhere—especially in the USA—forms a stock theme of official writing and the contrast serves to confirm the validity of a communist system. There is thus an in-built tendency to gloss over the fact that several types of health service charge are in operation on a uniform basis throughout the USSR.

The most readily identified of these charges is the payment for medicines consumed by out-patients (All in-patients are supplied with free drugs.) To call this a prescription charge would be misleading, since the same price is payable whether the drug has been prescribed in a course of treatment or is simply purchased across the counter. Moreover, it does not operate at a flat rate but varies with the drug in question. Prices do not necessarily reflect full production costs and are generally at a fairly low level.

Other health service charges relate to the dental and ophthalmic services and the supply of various types of prosthesis. Although a stay in hospital is always entirely free, residence at a sanatorium or health resort may entail direct payment by the patient.[11] At a theoretical level this practice might be justified on the ground that the treatments in question do not occupy a critical position in the range of health care. More directly relevant, however, is the point that trade union organizations frequently meet the costs in the case of individual workers, an arrangement which is closely linked with labour discipline and labour incentives.

The total sum disbursed by patients each year is not published, nor is the cost to the government budget of exempting certain groups from payment. Prominent among these are out-patients receiving treatment for one of a specified list of diseases. The list includes communicable diseases, such as tuberculosis, syphilis, dysentery and leprosy, in respect of which it is clearly desirable to ensure that patients are not debarred from following a course of treatment because of the cost of drugs. Also covered are chronic conditions, such as diabetes, cancer, schizophrenia and epilepsy, for which the cost of drugs could prove extremely burdensome over a period of time. Similarly no payment is made for drugs prescribed for children under one year of age. (In this respect the United Kingdom is far more generous since the health service prescription charge is not payable by children under the age of sixteen or by young persons under twenty-one still attending school on a full-time basis.) It is also the case that orthopaedic prostheses are supplied free to children and adolescents. All forms of prosthesis—dental, ophthalmic, and so on—are free to invalids of the Second World War and individuals in receipt of 'personal' pensions, which are distinct from ordinary pensions, being awarded for valued service to the state given by Party members and the like. These two groups also benefit from a reduction of eighty per cent on the cost of prescribed medicines and probably dressings as well.[12]

The account given above is taken from a source published in 1970 and it is possible, though not at all probable, that arrangements for exemption and price concessions have become more generous since that time. In this context mention should be made of the fact that the *Communist Party Programme*[13] of 1961 envisaged that the supply of medicines (and treatment of sick persons at sanatoria) would become free of charge by 1980. However, no subsequent reaffirmation of this policy has occurred as the date for its realization draws nearer. In the 1969 health service legislation the commitment was watered down to a vague reference to 'the gradual extension of curative means supplied free of charge or at a reduced rate...'.[14]

One explanation of this retreat could be that health planners consider that some payment by the majority of patients is desirable or essential in order to depress the demand for medicines. On a more general level, reference can be made to the less utopian or idealist priorities pursued by Soviet rulers in the period which has ensued since the fall from power of Nikita Krushchev.

So far as the author is aware, no public debate has occurred about the ideological propriety of health service charges—in marked contrast to the situation in Britain. Why has the issue not been raised? The answer is probably to be sought not so much in the power of the Party and government to 'screen out' discussion on embarrassing topics as in the comparative irrelevance of such a topic when the range and availability of drugs is so open to criticism. It is not difficult to amass a substantial body of published evidence on the shortcomings of the Soviet pharmaceutical industry and although real improvement has unquestionably occurred with the passage of time, production and distribution in this sector of the economy is still widely perceived as unsatisfactory.

PAYMENT AT TIME OF RECEIPT

In the Soviet Union, as can easily be inferred, official ideology is entirely hostile to the concept of a market in medical care. Indeed the existence in other countries of private practice on a large scale receives condemnation as a hallmark of bourgeois capitalist society where man exploits man and where, to quote a propaganda phrase, 'medicine is business'. An obvious institutional implication is that since the Revolution no private individual or autonomous group has been permitted to construct and equip premises designed specifically for the delivery of medical care. As a consequence, a wide range of diagnostic tests, operative procedures and regimes of treatment are obtainable only in state-controlled units.

Potential demand for private treatment has also been substantially reduced by another strategy: the provision of units which give preferential care to certain occupational groups and members of the Party and government elite. (More will be said about these units in chapter 8.) Less significant but having a comparable impact are the state-provided 'self-financing' polyclinics and nursing homes which form part of the main health service in urban areas. Although their numbers are nowhere recorded, Kaser has estimated that they probably total around 130 in the Soviet Union as a whole.[15]

From a Soviet source published in English, the following facts can be gleaned about these 'self-financing' units. For some patients they have the attraction of offering a free choice of doctor, which does not apply elsewhere. For others their consultancy function is paramount—a second opinion can be obtained from doctors with superior qualifications and more specialized experience who attend the clinics on a part-time basis. Patients are also attracted by the shorter waiting times for a consultation and some believe (erroneously, according to the source) that by paying they can obtain better-quality care.

As for the fees, these vary according to the qualifications of the doctor but in general are low. Thus in 1969 it was said to cost no more than two roubles—a little less than a pound—to consult a senior specialist. Ear, nose and throat operations cost from one to $2\frac{1}{2}$ roubles. However, it must be recognized that no cash nexus exists between doctor and patient; the latter makes his payment direct to the polyclinic. And after diagnosis has been established, a patient can receive the prescribed course of treatment at his usual polyclinic free of charge.[16]

While no documentary evidence has been found to support the point, it appears that certain forms of provision are obtainable only at these special facilities. On the basis of conversations with Russians, the author has certainly formed the impression that this applies in the case of dental treatment which is more expensive than necessary, and in the case of ophthalmic supplies other than the utility type. Similarly, patients seeking surgery on purely cosmetic grounds will have to enter a nursing home where payment is made. One further reason which has been given for attendance at pay polyclinics is that they offer conditions of greater anonymity for the patient presenting with a sexually transmitted disease.

Other institutional arrangements can be identified as elements in an overall policy calculated to force private practice into a highly marginal place. The process of hospitalization can take place only via the state service and there are no 'pay beds' for private patients such as obtain in the United Kingdom in a number of National

Health Service hospitals. Similarly the function of supplying sick-leave certificates is restricted to state polyclinics and other such units. In the past at any rate, the state also employed a crude form of suppression by harrassment and ideological barrage, to judge from a passage in Alexander Solzhenitsin's novel *Cancer Ward*. One of the characters in it is an elderly doctor named Dormidont Tikhono-vich Oreshchenkov, and his experience during the 1920s and 1930s is described as follows:

> ... among all these persecutions the most persistent and oppressive had been on account of the fact that Oreshchenkov stubbornly insisted on his right to run a private medical practice although it was everywhere forbidden with increasing severity as a source of private enterprise and enrichment and as an activity divorced from honest work which at every turn and every day fostered the emergence of a bourgeoisie. There were several years when he had to take down his brass plate and turn away every patient no matter how much they implored him and no matter how ill they were, because the neighbourhood was full of spies, voluntary and paid, from the tax office and because the patients themselves could not stop themselves gossiping about their treatment. And this led to the doctor being threatened with the loss of all his work [he also held a salaried post], even with the loss of his house.
>
> Nevertheless it was precisely his right to run a private practice that he valued above all in his calling ...[17]

At the time of writing, it appears that active repression has given way to discouragement by means of administrative regulation, in particular by high rates of tax on income earned from private practice. But a training in medicine endows its recipient with an inalienable basis of knowledge and personal skills. Although the Soviet Union may have adopted all practical steps to bring the doctor–patient relationship under the state aegis to maximum extent, there can be no doubt of the prevalence of personalized money transactions between patient and doctor. Openly acknowledged and administratively separate private practice has been reduced to a what is probably a negligible level, but unofficial payment is commonplace for services provided ostensibly under the state scheme.

Evidence of this practice is by no means hard to obtain. For example, Hendrick Smith reports that 'A workman told me he had paid 50 rubles ($66) to the surgeon in a state hospital for operating on his legs after he fell down an elevator shaft, and a chauffeur said he paid 150 rubles to have three of his wife's teeth capped'.[18] Kaser was even able to publish an unofficial tariff of charges for various types of service.[19]

It must be added that the tipping of nurses and orderlies can be an ordinary and perhaps unavoidable concomitant of a stay in hospital. That was certainly true for one resident of Odessa whose experience was recently reported in *Izvestiya*. Suffering from acute appendicitis, citizen K asked his wife to put a good supply of one-rouble notes in his pocket before the ambulance came. On arrival at the city's emergency care hospital, the attendants simply got out and walked away. At length K bargained with a man in a white coat who, with the aid of a companion, carried him to the operating theatre for two roubles. During convalescence K received good treatment because he tipped generously, but eventually his notes were used up and he had to wait a long time for everything—injections, thermometers, a glass of water, even the bedpan. After his wife had replenished the supply of money, the former efficiency returned. At this hospital, wrote *Izvestiya*'s correspondent, the orderlies 'will not even lift a finger without direct material stimulus on the part of the patients'.[20]

It is only proper to add that unofficial payment is widespread in many sectors of what is still a far from consumer-oriented society. Whether the practice is any more prevalent in the health service than elsewhere is a question for which no answer can be offered. However, there is no reason to overlook the fact that the salaries of medical staff may help to foster or at least do nothing to inhibit payments intended to secure more prompt and better-quality treatment. The comparatively low salaries received by doctors is one of the themes which will be pursued in the next chapter.

CHAPTER 3

The Supply of Doctors

One of the factors which are clearly critical for the organization of medical care is an adequate supply of health service personnel in general and of doctors in particular. In the Soviet Union, as is fairly well-known, social and economic development has been accompanied by a rapid growth in the number of doctors. By the end of 1974 the total had reached 799,000, which represents a truly massive achievement, even taking account of the fact that the term doctor also embraces two grades of dentist. A threefold increase had occurred since 1950, the earliest post-war year for which such data are published.

When the absolute figures are related to the population of the USSR, an altered but still impressive picture emerges. In 1950, as Table 3.1 shows, there were 14.6 doctors for every 10,000 inhabitants and by the end of 1974 the ratio stood at 31.5 per 10,000, having more than doubled over this period. For a number of years the Soviet government has made considerable propaganda use of its doctor-to-population ratios since they rank very high in international comparisons. Indeed in this respect the Soviet Union stands well ahead of all other economically developed nations, with the exception of Israel. (See Appendix 3 for data from selected countries.)

Notwithstanding the already generous supply of doctors, a further very substantial increase has been projected for the future. In January 1973 the USSR Ministry of Health published a norm in connection with the tenth five-year plan which set the ideal long-term ratio at 38.2 per 10,000 persons.[1] As it happens, this norm was cited in a publication by a leading health service planner who, only a few years earlier, had stated that the ideal ratio had been

34

fixed at 34.6 doctors per 10,000 total population.[2] The discrepancy here is perhaps most cogently explained simply by postulating that a sizeable upward revision of the estimated demand for doctors came to be accepted as necessary. Apparently no date has been specified for the achievement of the norm, and it is intended[3] that a ratio of 35.7 per 10,000 should be achieved by the year 1980.

TABLE 3.1   *Number of doctors, 1950–1974*

| | End of years: | | | |
	1950	1960	1970	1974
Number	265,000	431,700	668,400	799,000
Doctors per 10,000 population	14.6	20.0	27.4	31.5

Notes: (a) Doctors in the armed forces are explicitly excluded from the figures for 1950 and 1960 and are probably excluded from the figures for 1970 and 1974.

     (b) Following the Soviet practice, two grades of dentist are included.

Sources: *Narodnoe Khozyaistvo SSSR* for 1965, p. 744; and for 1974, p. 728.

As might easily be inferred from what has been said, the Soviet Union contains a large number of higher educational establishments for medical training. These consist of nine medical faculties attached to universities and eighty-three separate medical institutes, which exemplify the Soviet preference for locating applied studies in single-purpose as opposed to multi-purpose establishments. On successful completion of his course, the young doctor will receive a diploma, not a degree, even if he has attended a university.

The size of annual intakes must clearly be substantial. For the academic year starting in 1975, the new students numbered about 57,000 and, according to the Health Minister, admissions will stabilize at this level.[4] Perhaps about ten per cent are foreign nationals, the vast majority of whom come from developing countries. It might be supposed that the sheer size of the intake means that less individual instruction is provided than in a British medical school, but evidence is not available to prove the point.

SPATIAL VARIATION

Thus far reference has been made to data for the USSR as a whole and it is essential to recognize that doctor-to-population ratios vary quite considerably as between the fifteen Union republics. This point is brought out in Table 3.2, which gives figures for the years 1950 and 1974. In both years Georgia came first in rank order, while the

TABLE 3.2   *Number of doctors by Union republic in 1950 and 1974*

Republic	End of 1950		End of 1974	
	Absolute number	Doctors per 10,000 persons	Absolute number	Doctors per 10,000 persons
RSFSR	160,200	15.6	451,100	33.7
Ukrainian SSR	51,700	13.9	150,800	30.9
Belorussian SSR	7,200	9.3	27,400	29.4
Uzbek SSR	6,600	10.2	33,400	24.4
Kazakh SSR	6,400	9.5	37,100	26.2
Georgian SSR	9,500	26.7	19,100	38.8
Azerbaidzhan SSR	6,400	22.0	15,500	27.6
Lithuanian SSR	2,800	10.7	10,800	32.9
Moldavian SSR	2,500	10.3	9,500	24.9
Latvian SSR	2,900	15.1	9,500	38.3
Kirgiz SSR	1,800	9.9	7,800	23.6
Tadzhik SSR	1,300	8.4	6,600	19.6
Armenian SSR	2,600	18.9	9,200	33.0
Turkmen SSR	1,600	13.4	6,100	24.4
Estonian SSR	1,500	13.5	5,100	36.0

Sources: *Narodnoe Khozyaistvo SSSR* for 1970, p. 690; and for 1974, p. 728.

Central Asian republic of Tadzhikistan came bottom. It is noteworthy that although the latter more than doubled its ratio from 8.4 to 19.6 doctors per 10,000 persons over this period, it failed to narrow the gap with Georgia. The range in fact increased slightly from 18.3 to 19.2 doctors per 10,000 persons.

In the past, a proportion of newly qualified doctors were directed to work in republics other than those in which they trained. A study published in 1963 stated that although this practice had proved valuable, it resulted in a high turn-over rate; on completion of their three years' compulsory service, the young doctors normally returned to their parents' place of domicile or to the town in which they trained. From about 1962–3, according to this source, individual republics were intended to rely on the output of their own medical institutes, at least for doctors practising curative medicine. It has not been possible to establish when—and indeed whether—the inter-republic direction of doctors was discontinued.

During the 1950s a number of new training establishments were brought into commission to help boost the supply of doctors in Central Asia and Siberia, among other places. By 1960 the USSR had eighty medical institutes and five medical faculties at universities, with at least one training establishment for each republic, however small its population. In the same year the number of students per thousand population, a key index, was above the all-Union average in the Kazakh and Kirgiz republics and well above it in Turkmenia and Uzbekistan. Clearly a determined effort was being mounted to achieve a higher than average output of newly qualified doctors in these under-supplied republics.[5]

DOCTORS FOR THE BACKWOODS

Marked variations in the supply of doctors occur not only between republics but also between urban and rural areas within them. In 1974 the main health service possessed 34.5 doctors per 10,000 urban population, but only 17.9 per 10,000 rural population—even taking into account the staff in urban institutions which admit patients from the countryside. The rural areas in a few republics such as Tadzhikistan and Kirgizia had significantly lower ratios than the all-Union average.[6]

The problem of ensuring that rural areas have sufficient doctors is one that has long preoccupied the authorities and it has not yet been resolved, despite heavy reliance on a form of direction of labour. The author has been unable to obtain a precise description of the institutional arrangements currently in force but is under the impression that the medical institutes, having been informed of vacant posts in their regions and perhaps elsewhere, are required to register individual students for specific posts. In theory these must be held for three years commencing immediately after the period of internship, which takes place in a large urban hospital. There appears to be a degree of choice for the students, at least to the extent that the academically ablest are given an opportunity to opt for more attractive vacancies located in urban areas.

Compulsory service in the rural backwoods is presented as an obligation incumbent on a young doctor and the oath which is now taken on qualification includes the promise 'to work conscientiously in the place demanded by the interests of society'. (For the full text of this oath see Appendix 4.) Whatever the force of moral suasion, however, it is clear that many doctors successfully evade their posting to the country. A recent study relating to the Mogilev and Brest regions of Belorussia reported that twenty to thirty per cent of interns never arrived at their destinations. It continued: 'During the year of work in a large town many changes in one's life can occur. And so a doctor alters the itinerary which was arranged earlier on account of "family reasons" or other obstacles.'[7] As for the reference to 'family reasons', presumably marriage is regarded as a sufficient justification for cancellation of the posting in the case of women doctors.

Another aspect of the problem is the reluctance of doctors to remain in remoter rural settings once their compulsory service has been completed. The extent of this 'instability of cadres' in the recent past was indicated by one of the Union's deputy Health Ministers. In 1967 he wrote that each year about forty per cent of newly qualified doctors were directed to take up posts in the country, the absolute number being about 63,000 doctors over the years 1959–65. But the net gain was small, on account of a high return rate, with about 55,000 leaving for urban areas over the same period. 'In many republics', the Minister stated, 'up to forty per cent of doctors who work in a rural area—and in the Turkmen republic 42.8 per cent—have less than four years' length of service.'[8] It seems highly probable that the situation has improved little, if at all, since that time.

A variety of factors can be identified as influencing young doctors to return to urban areas as soon as possible. Among them are the difficulty of obtaining satisfactory living quarters and the socio-cultural advantages enjoyed by the urban population. These alone may more than nullify the effect of inducements to remain, the more tangible of which are a somewhat higher pay scale and earlier age for retirement. From a career viewpoint also there are compelling reasons for returning; these centre on the fact that Soviet medical practice is dominated by specialization, and advancement as a specialist is ruled out for the one doctor on the staff of a small sector hospital. In the past, at any rate, this situation has been compounded by the difficulty of practising modern medicine in some of these small units. Here it is relevant to quote from an article published by *Meditsinskaya Gazeta* in 1964 which censured the director of the Orenburg regional health department in the following words:

> Let us take up the fundamental question—the problem of the place of work. In the Orenburg region it is related in many cases to the 'dwarf' hospitals. Have they really not yet understood here that if the sector hospital has only ten to fifteen beds (and there are sixty-seven such hospitals in the region), if there is no laboratory or X-ray equipment and the hospital is far from the district centre, then it is not possible in such conditions to organize a good medical service for the population. Could a doctor be retained here?[9]

At the time of writing, it is clear that there is no likelihood of phasing out compulsory service in the foreseeable future. In fact larger numbers of young doctors are now being directed to the countryside. With improvements in living conditions and in the organization of rural medical care, the problem of 'instability' may become less acute, but it is most unlikely to disappear.

STAFF POSTS

The large net increase in the number of doctors has been predicated upon planned expansion in medical manpower requirements. In this context a key concept is the 'staff post' (which relates to paramedical workers in addition to doctors). According to Dr G. A. Popov, the number of posts required is determined by reference to: (1) norms for hours of work; (2) workload norms; (3) staffing standards which have been worked out both for the Union as a whole and for specific types of institution and administrative units.[10]

As could be predicted, not all posts for doctors are actually occupied. In 1974 there was a total of 839,000 staff posts for doctors in the medico–sanitary institutions of the main health service, but only 798,610 were filled. The average value of the 'index of manning' stood at 95.2 per cent and varied from ninety-two per cent in Tadzhikistan to 99.7 per cent in Latvia. The index also reveals variations as between units located in urban and in rural areas. The average for the former was 95.9 per cent, with a range running from 93.4 per cent in Tadzhikistan to 99.5 in Estonia. The all-Union average for rural institutions was 88.8 per cent, with 80.5 per cent in Armenia and 96.7 per cent in Latvia.

It should be added that the number of posts occupied is related to the extent to which doctors hold a second appointment. The opportunity to occupy a second post (which may be in another specialty) is frequently referred to in announcements of vacant positions which are published by *Meditsinskaya Gazeta*, but it is not clear whether a doctor can be required to avail himself of the opportunity. In the main health service in 1974 the 'coefficient of pluralism' stood at 1.22—that is to say, there were 1.22 occupied posts to every one doctor. For urban institutions the average coefficient was 1.21, with values ranging from 1.1 in Armenia to 1.39 in the Tadzhik republic. A significantly less favourable situation existed in rural areas where the average was 1.34 and the range ran from 1.19 in Estonia to 1.48 in Tadzhikistan.[11] Making the main point in a different way, relatively more rural doctors hold two posts.

A breakdown of occupied posts in the main health service for the years 1965 and 1974 provides further evidence of the persisting imbalance between urban and rural areas—as well as giving an indication of how posts are distributed within the system. From Table 3.3 it can be seen that occupied posts connected with the curative–prophylactic service for the rural population increased from 125,890 to 166,120 during this period (the figures include posts in urban institutions which admit patients from rural areas). But a much larger proportional increase occurred in respect of urban services—the number of posts rose sharply from 373,000 in 1965 to 549,980 in 1974. It is appropriate to add that the development of specialized departments in larger hospitals has had some bearing on the differential growth rate.

TABLE 3.3 *Posts for doctors in main health service in 1965 and 1974*

Section of health service	Number of occupied posts		Occupied posts per 10,000 population	
	1965	1974	1965	1974
Out-patient care for urban population	264,200	397,940	21.18	25.98
Out-patient care for rural population provided in towns	27,930	44,090	2.39	4.40
Hospital care for urban population	108,800	152,040	8.72	9.92
Hospital care for rural population provided in towns	36,460	50,270	3.11	5.02
Curative–prophylactic care in rural areas	61,500	71,760	5.25	7.17
Total curative–prophylactic care for urban population	373,000	549,980	29.90	35.90
Total curative–prophylactic care for rural population	125,890	166,120	10.75	16.59
Psychiatric and psycho-neurological hospitals	10,610	16,880	0.46	0.67
Children's homes, homes for mothers and children	1,390	1,370	0.06	0.05
Sanatoria	10,490	12,030	0.45	0.47
Environmental health institutions	31,620	47,490	1.36	1.88
Bureaux of forensic-medical expertise	3,070	4,740	0.13	0.19
Total posts in medico-sanitary system	561,520	798,610	24.22	31.53
Scientific research institutes, higher and intermediate educational establishments, administration of health service organs	40,200	63,840	1.73	2.52
TOTAL NUMBER OF POSTS	601,720	862,450	25.95	34.05
COEFFICIENT OF PLURALISM	1.25	1.22		
TOTAL NUMBER OF DOCTORS	483,100	708,090	20.84	27.96

Source: Popov, *Ekonomika i planirovanie zdravookhraneniya*, p. 277.

A PREPONDERANCE OF WOMEN

One of the most striking features about Soviet medical cadres is that women form such a sizeable proportion of the total complement. This phenomenon is by no means of recent origin; large numbers of women were being admitted to medical institutes in the immediate post-Revolutionary period. Even as early as 1923, according to G. A. Popov, equality had been achieved in the sex ratio among newly qualified doctors in the Russian republic.[12] The proportion of women doctors increased rapidly during the inter-war years to reach an all-Union average of sixty-two per cent in 1940.

The manpower strategies which were employed during the Second World War entailed an even higher proportion of women among the annual intakes at medical institutes. As a consequence, by 1950 women accounted for seventy-seven per cent of the total number of Soviet civilian doctors. They had also constituted a very sizeable proportion, perhaps about a half, of all service doctors during the war.

Since that time the pendulum has swung back to a small extent; according to official data the proportion of women among qualified doctors had fallen to seventy-two per cent by 1970 and was at seventy per cent by the end of 1975.[13] Although the author has been unable to establish precise sex ratios in medical institutes and faculties, an approximate assessment is possible on the basis of surrogate data.[14] It can be suggested that the proportion of women in the medical student population declined from sixty-five per cent at the start of the academic year 1950/51 to fifty-six per cent ten years later but had fallen no further by 1975/6. It is interesting that the figure is not lower, given the discrimination in favour of male applicants to medical institutes which takes the form of setting the pass mark in entrance examinations at a lower level for men.

The figures cited above relate to the whole Union but they do not conceal very marked variations between individual republics. The latest breakdown by republics which the author has obtained relates to 1966 and reveals that, at the end of the year, the percentages ranged from sixty in Tadzhikistan and Turkmenia to seventy-nine in Latvia.[15] It is frequently emphasized that women doctors now figure prominently even in those areas of Imperial Russia whose social and economic development had been least advanced.

The sex ratio does reveal variation, however, from one specialty to another. This point can be proved for Armenia, and there is no sound reason for supposing that the picture should be markedly different in other republics. According to data cited by Popov, which probably relate to the mid- or late-1960s, the percentages ranged from 94.4 for paediatricians to 20.2 for surgeons. The physically demanding nature of surgery is perhaps the most cogent explanation for male dominance in this specialty. Special considerations can also be adduced for the fact that men outnumbered women in radiology and dermato-venereology as well.[16]

As for promotion prospects, considerable significance attaches to the fact that women hold a quite disproportionately small number of senior positions in the medical hierarchy. One Soviet economist, writing in 1969, drew attention to the anomaly that although men accounted for only fifteen per cent of the medical workforce, they occupied half the posts for chief doctors and directors of medical institutions.[17] In 1975 none of the Union republics had a female Health Minister, although it should be added that eleven women doctors held appointments as deputy Ministers of Union republics while three were Health Ministers in autonomous republics. As for the academic and research fields, in the same year six women were rectors of medical institutes and institutes for advanced training while thirty-seven held the post of director of a scientific research establishment.[18] Only one woman has succeeded in reaching the top of the medico-administrative pyramid; M. D. Kovrigina was Union Minister of Health from 1954 to 1959.

The preponderance of women in the medical workforce could be held to reflect that abolition of discrimination on grounds of sex which, formally at least, occurred in the early days of the Bolshevik government. A far more powerful explanatory factor, however, is the relative lack of importance assigned to the service sector of the economy. It is difficult to disagree with Mark Field's judgment that 'in view of the overall personnel shortages in the economy and the high priority commitment to industrialization and to tasks *directly* relevant to this process, it may be fair to say that the impressive increases in the size of the medical group could not have taken place without the large-scale employment of women in medicine'.[19]

Official propaganda certainly emphasizes the natural suitability of women for this caring vocation and it seems that many young people in the Soviet Union have a stereotyped image of medicine as an occupation mainly for women. However that may be, working conditions make it relatively easy for a married woman to combine employment in this field with the responsibilities of a wife and mother. Thus the professional obligations of doctor providing primary care end with the completion of her shift at the polyclinic and she will not be 'on call' at home. Moreover, a sizeable proportion of doctors put in no more than $5\frac{1}{2}$ hours per day in a five-day week. This is a point for which allowance should be made when comparing the doctor-to-population ratios in the Soviet Union on one hand and most Western countries on the other.

A further observation which should be made in this context is that the preponderance of women constitutes one of the influences which serve to reduce differentiation between doctors and para-medical workers. At this point the discussion verges on questions of socio-occupational status, and further progress in that direction would be beyond the scope of this study. However, it would be unduly restrictive not to report the view about the sex ratio expressed by certain Soviet doctors to a visting delegation from the USA. On the basis of discussions at the First Moscow Medical Institute and possibly elsewhere, this delegation recorded that 'Many administrators and faculty members stated the ideal ratio would be thirty per cent women and seventy per cent men, since women have difficulty raising families while doing professional work'.[20] In comment it must be said that the major obstacle to the achievement of this ideal is the relatively low financial rewards which Soviet doctors receive.

SALARIES

Those individuals who obtain high positions in the academic or bureaucratic hierarchies probably receive very substantial incomes, but the majority of their colleagues are certainly far from well paid by Soviet standards. According to *Narodnoe Khozyaistvo SSSR*, in 1972 the average monthly salary for manual and white-collar workers was 130.2 roubles.[21] In September of that year, doctors received what was apparently their first pay increase since 1964 and under the new regulations staff with a work record of up to five years were to receive from 100 to 145 roubles per month, depending on the nature of the post. For those with thirty or more years' service, the top of the salary scale varies from 170 to 180 roubles per month.[22]

No data are available to indicate the number of doctors who actually receive salaries below the national average and, as was shown above, there are considerable opportunities to hold a second post and thus increase take-home pay. That there are real financial pressures to do so was suggested by one set of findings from a large-scale survey undertaken in the Russian Republic in 1968. The survey revealed that the holding of more than one post declined with an increase in family income divided by the number of persons dependent on it. Thus where family income per person was below sixty roubles per month, 62.3 per cent of the doctors held two jobs, but where it was eighty to ninety-nine roubles per month only 44.3 per cent had a second post.[23]

Wasteful Deployment of Doctors

Given the existence of relatively low salaries, there is likely to be little incentive to conserve a doctor's time strictly for those tasks—diagnosing, advising and treating patients—which are central to the medical function. That the skills of Soviet doctors were far from being conserved had become a cause of concern to health bureaucrats by about 1963–4 and attention focussed on methods of preventing the 'irrational' use of a doctor's time. The extent of gross wastefulness was thrown into sharp relief by a range of investigations carried out during the late-1960s by the N. A. Semashko Institute of Social Hygiene and Organization of Medical Care. Thus the report of one work-study, carried out in four industrial towns, revealed that forty out-patient doctors in the main specialties had 'reserves of time' which totalled between fifteen and fifty per cent of their available man-hours, depending on the specialty. The report recommended revising a number of 'orders, instructions and regulations' concerning the organization of out-patient work, with precedence being given to the regulations concerning certification of lack of fitness for work.[24] Similarly, a survey of ear, nose and throat specialists in polyclinics, undertaken not long afterwards, revealed that about thirty per cent of these doctors' day was expended on various types of activity such as meetings, documentation and administrative problems which had no immediate bearing on the diagnosis and treatment of patients.[25]

Investigations such as the ones cited above form one aspect of the wider field of activity known as the scientific organization of work, which has clearly had a significant impact on the health service in recent years. Among the more obvious changes evident to a returning visitor is the widespread introduction of mechanical aids, such as dictaphones, which significantly reduce the amount of time devoted to medical documentation. It is unclear whether a reduction has taken place in the amount of certification required from a doctor.

A highly relevant question to which little attention has been devoted is the possibility of reallocating some of a doctor's functions to less highly trained personnel. That there is scope for redefining the job description—certainly in one specialty—emerges from a study intended to elucidate the low popularity of posts in environmental health. Out of 400 doctors employed within this area of activity who replied to a postal questionnaire in 1966, a significant proportion—twenty-eight per cent—stated that they were dissatisfied with their work. In response to the question: 'How, in your opinion, should the work of an environmental health doctor be rationalized?', 18.5 per cent said that they should be freed from work which was below their competence while 13.6 per cent recommended an increase in the number of environmental health assistants.[26] The present writer has no evidence as to whether doctors who have clinical responsibility for patients also consider that some of their work could be reallocated, but he has formed the impression that certain procedures undertaken by doctors in the USSR would be performed by nurses in Britain.

Here it is relevant to add that, by comparison with Britain, the Soviet Union has a more restricted range of groups in health care and related fields. Thus there is no equivalent to our social worker —an omission which is probably best explained by reference to ideological difficulties which would flow from acceptance of the concept of social work. Similarly no counterpart can be found for the professionally-trained lay administrators who play a key role in the management of the British health service. That omission may reflect a comparative lack of emphasis on managerial and administrative skills as much as the lack of a financial incentive to substitute laymen for doctors in respect of non-clinical functions.

At the start of this chapter it was implied that the doctor-to-population ratio obtaining in the Soviet Union was substantially more generous than those of Western countries. It is now possible to conclude that this achievement has necessarily entailed rejection of the Western pattern of a highly remunerated and male-dominated profession. The Soviet strategy has depended for its success on the mutually reinforcing factors of relatively low pay and a large proportion of women doctors.

CHAPTER 4

Specialization in Medicine

It is arguable that the Soviet Union would not need to achieve such very high doctor-to-population ratios but for the heavy emphasis placed on specialization. This constitutes a feature of medical practice which official pronouncements frequently refer to and which no account of the system should neglect. Of course there are problems of definition to take into account and at the outset it must be made clear that the word 'specialist' in this chapter will not be used in the British sense of a hospital-based doctor to whom patients are referred by their generalist family practitioner. But the wide connotation of the word in Russian in no way invalidates the point that specialization plays a key part in the theoretical underpinning of the Soviet health service.

The reason for its prominence resides in an unqualified acceptance of the view that medico–scientific knowledge and skills have developed to a point where specialization has become essential for practising clinicians. A succinct but authoritative statement of the official doctrine on the score was made a few years ago by the Union's Health Minister. He said: 'Specialization in respect of general medical, surgical and other forms of medical care is essential since it is impossible to conceive that only a single doctor with a broad background could fully guarantee highly qualified care for patients suffering from a variety of illnesses which are frequently complicated to diagnose and treat'.[1]

THE BROAD DIVISIONS

While specialization is to be expected at postgraduate level, in the Soviet Union it begins even during initial training at medical institute. In place of the single entry to practice, long familiar in Britain and other countries, the USSR has created a number of gateways which lead into different branches of medicine. Far from following a generic course, intending doctors train separately for the following broad fields: environmental health, paediatrics, stomatology (dental surgery) and what is termed curative medicine.

Within most medical institutes there can be found separate faculties covering the above-mentioned fields and on entry, apparently, students commit themselves to one of the broad divisions. Institutes do not necessarily contain all faculties and some, as their titles indicate, focus solely on one branch of medicine. Examples are the Moscow Stomatological Institute and the recently completed Central Asian Institute of Paediatric Medicine. Although faculties of military medicine are located in certain civilian institutes, single-purpose establishments also exist for training service doctors.

During the last decade, relatively small numbers of students have been admitted to newly created faculties for the training of bio-medical research scientists. These personnel do not have clinical responsibility for patients and are probably excluded from the official records of the number of doctors. Some medical institutes also contain pharmaceutical faculties, though the majority of pharmacists qualify after a shorter training in the intermediate-level institutes. It is also in the latter that courses are provided for 'dental practitioners', the second grade of dentist.

Some degree of overlap in course-content undoubtedly exists between the different types of basic medical education and must be quite considerable in paediatrics and curative medicine. The separation of these two areas of work at undergraduate level may appear puzzling, even when allowance is made for the Soviet emphasis on specialization. From the range of health service policies and institutions, however, it can be deduced that the explanation lies not so much in the knowledge-bases of these two divisions as in the special priority which the government has assigned to health care for the citizens and workforce of tomorrow. This priority is manifest in the existence of units catering solely for child patients; it can also be seen as the rationale behind separate undergraduate training in paediatrics and the large proportion of doctors absorbed by this specialty.

Whatever the precise extent of the common element in different courses, significant numbers of doctors have been obliged to practise in a basic division other than the one in which they qualified. This form of resource substitution has caused most concern where stomatologists and environmental health doctors are concerned. In the early 1960s a Western commentator, who was probably quoting Soviet sources, reported that in many areas the health authorities called upon twenty-five to thirty per cent of stomatologists to work in one or other field of curative medicine.[2] Since that time, such stop-gap action has declined owing to increased output of appropriately qualified cadres—and to official prohibition. Thus in 1971 the Union Health Minister declared: 'It is necessary to put a decisive end to the erroneous practice of using environmental health doctors in curative work'.[3]

BROAD AND NARROW SPECIALTIES

A more detailed breakdown of medical cadres is presented in the statistical yearbook; there the overwhelming majority of doctors are assigned to one or other of the fifteen so-called basic specialties. Four of the entries are accounted for by groupings already mentioned: paediatricians, environmental health doctors, stomatologists and dental practitioners. Taken together, these accounted for 30.1 per cent of the total in 1974. All the remaining specialties must represent basic subdivisions of curative medicine.

From Table 4.1 it is possible to compare the numbers assigned to the basic specialties in 1950 and 1974. As might be predicted, having regard to developments in medical science, surgeons have increased at an above-average rate and accounted for 10.2 per cent of the total at the end of the period compared with 8.5 per cent at the start. Substantial gains were made by otorhinolaryngologists (ear, nose and throat specialists), neuropathologists, psychiatrists, radiographers and radiologists and—most impressive of all—by stomatologists. The relative standing of environmental health doctors declined considerably, although it should be noted that they still accounted for 5.9 per cent of the total in 1974 and there is abundant evidence of a continuing concern to develop facilities in this field. Specialists in tuberculosis also lost ground, but the fact that they still outnumbered psychiatrists in 1974 makes a remarkable comment on medical needs and priorities in the Soviet Union of today.

In both 1950 and 1974, the second largest group consisted of a residual category, the existence of which becomes evident only when

TABLE 4.1   *Doctors by main specialty in 1950 and 1974*

Specialty	End of 1950		End of 1974	
	Number	%	Number	%
General physicians*	56,000	21.1	164,800	20.6
Surgeons†	22,500	8.5	81,700	10.2
Obstetricians–gynaecologists	16,600	6.3	47,400	5.9
Paediatricians	32,100	12.1	91,500	11.5
Ophthalmologists	5,700	2.2	17,400	2.2
Otorhinolaryngologists	4,600	1.7	17,500	2.2
Neuropathologists	5,100	1.9	20,500	2.6
Psychiatrists	3,100	1.2	17,700	2.2
Specialists in tuberculosis	9,400	3.5	23,100	2.9
Dermato-venereologists	9,200	3.5	14,100	1.8
Radiologists and radio-therapists	6,200	2.3	27,900	3.5
Specialists in physical culture and sport	800	0.3	3,900	0.5
Doctors of the sanitary and anti-epidemic group‡	21,900	8.3	47,300	5.9
Stomatologists	10,400	3.9	51,500	6.4
Dental practitioners	17,700	6.7	50,100	6.3
Residual group§	43,700	16.5	122,600	15.3
TOTAL	265,000	100	799,000	100

* Includes specialists in physiotherapy, endocrinology and infectious diseases.

† Includes specialists in traumatology and orthopaedics, oncology, anaesthetics and reanimation, and urology.

‡ Includes specialists in sanitation, epidemiology, bacteriology and virology and disinfectionists.

§ Not given in source; obtained by subtracting numbers listed under each specialty from the grand total.

Sources: *Narodnoe Khozyaistvo SSSR* for 1970, p. 691; and for 1974, p. 729.

the numbers given under each specialty are subtracted from the total. Who then are these unidentified personnel? In 1974, though not in 1950, some of them were young doctors still completing their medical training as interns. Medical administrators and, in all probability, doctors employed in forensic–medical institutions are also assigned to this category.

It is also evident, on *a priori* grounds, that the specialist groups exclude staff occupying posts which are formally designated for 'doctors of general practice'. These posts exist in health points and emergency aid stations of small towns and, more particularly, in the smallest rural hospitals. Notwithstanding the fact that the staff in question will have trained in one of the broad divisions, they can be termed generalists quite appropriately since many of them have to provide as full a range of diagnosis and treatment as possible for a population of patients which is undifferentiated by age, sex or disease category. But such a situation, far from being endorsed by conventional wisdom as in the United Kingdom, is tolerated only to the extent that it is unavoidable. In fact, the increasing stress on specialized medical care has been accompanied by a sizeable reduction in the number of general practitioners. This point can be illustrated by reference to the RSFSR where in 1950 they made up 6.9 per cent of doctors domiciled in towns and 20.3 per cent of those in rural areas. (The data relate only to the main health service and exclude dental doctors.) But by 1967 the figures had dropped to 2.7 and 12.9 per cent respectively.[4]

As the notes for Table 4.1 indicate, some of the fifteen basic specialties contain subdivisions, and this indication of differentiation points to a development of major significance. In recent decades and more especially since 1960, medicine in the Soviet Union has been subject to a process of fission whereby 'narrow' specialties have split off from 'broad' ones such as general medicine and surgery. (Of course this process is not unique to the Soviet Union even though it may have proceeded further there than in most other countries.) Thus the numbers entered under surgery also cover specialists in traumatology and orthopaedics, anaesthetics and reanimation, oncology, and urology.

But the propagation of new specialties has proceeded a good deal further than the table indicates. Sometimes newly designated areas of interest are in effect thrust upon the medical world, as was the case with the exogenous demands for skills in space medicine and in what is termed radiation hygiene. In general, however, the establishment of posts in new fields results from the decisions of influential clinicians and administrators within the service. It is interesting that the arguments for and against a new development may be openly debated in the medical press. One recent example relates to anaesthetics and reanimation; it is currently being established as a clinical discipline in its own right, and the pattern which this 'young specialty' should follow formed the subject of correspondence in *Meditsinskaya Gazeta* during 1975. The development of a separate service for children was advocated by a professor of paediatric surgery who took the view that 'Many specialists in adult anaesthetics and reanimation do not have an adequate understanding of the special anatomical features of a child and the doses of medicine and volume of infusion therapy appropriate for a given age; they are not familiar with the specifics of paediatric anaesthesiology'.[5]

That assertion raises the question whether the demarcation of one specialist area automatically creates pressures for the designation of another in some ever-expanding process. But more pertinent from the organizational viewpoint is the danger of specialization being taken so far that it gives rise to excessively compartmentalized activity and a blinkered perception of the patient. That such a risk was indeed recognized by Soviet doctors in the mid-1950s is suggested by a passage in Solzhenitsin's *Cancer Ward*. One of the characters, Ludmila Afanasyevna Donstova, 'was among the last doctors with a grasp of both x-ray diagnosis and x-ray therapy and despite the trend of the times towards the fragmentation of knowledge she attempted to ensure that her housemen kept up with the two'.[6] If that evidence is considered open to objection, no question can be raised concerning the authority of a comment made by a leading medical academic about the draft of the 1969 health service legislation. Professor Yu. Lisitsin wrote: '...it appears to be not entirely appropriate to place special emphasis on the all-embracing development of specialized medical care since at present there is a tendency towards a form of super-specialization that cannot fail to cause harm to the development of the basic medical specialties'.[7] Although conveyed in a subdued tone, that adds up to a fairly stringent criticism of the existing trend.

TABLE 4.2   *Nomenclature of medical specialists and territorial level of their employment*

	Specialty	Level of employment		
		Rural medical sector	*Institutions of a rural district*	*Remaining institutions*
1	General physician	+	+	+
2	Cardiorheumatologist		+	+
3	Gastroenterologist			+
4	Nephrologist			+
5	Endocrinologist		+	+
6	Haematologist			+
7	Specialist in infectious diseases	+	+	+
8	Dietician		+	+
9	Physiotherapist		+	+
10	Specialist in curative physical culture and sport		+	+
11	General physician in clinical physiology (electrocardiography and functional diagnosis)		+	+
12	Surgeon	+	+	+
13	Paediatric surgeon		+	+
14	Traumatologist–orthopaedist		+	+
15	Urologist		+	+
16	Neurosurgeon			+
17	Anaesthesiologist–reanimationist		+	+
18	Cardiovascular surgeon			+
19	Thoracic surgeon			+
20	Oncologist		+	+
21	Oncological surgeon		+	+
22	Oncological gynaecologist		+	+
23	Oncological otorhinolaryngologist		+	+
24	Oncological radiologist		+	+
25	Stomatologist	+	+	+
26	Stomatological surgeon			+
27	Stomatological orthopaedist		+	+
28	Obstetrician–gynaecologist	+	+	+
29	Paediatrician	+	+	+
30	Radiologist	+	+	+
31	Ophthalmologist		+	+
32	Paediatric ophthalmologist			+
33	Otorhinolaryngologist		+	+
34	Specialist in tuberculosis		+	+
35	Neuropathologist		+	+
36	Psychiatrist		+	+
37	Dermato-venereologist		+	+
38	Pathologist–anatomist		+	+
39	Toxicologist			+
40	Laboratory specialist		+	+

TABLE 4.2—*cont.*

Specialty	Level of employment		
	Rural medical sector	Institutions of a rural district	Remaining institutions
41 Forensic-medical specialist		+	+
42 Specialist in general hygiene		+	+
43 Specialist in communal hygiene		+	+
44 Specialist in occupational hygiene		+	+
45 Specialist in food hygiene		+	+
46 Specialist in the hygiene of children and adolescents		+	+
47 Specialist in radiation hygiene			+
48 Epidemiologist (disinfectionist, parasitologist)		+	+
49 Bacteriologist (virologist)		+	+
50 Social hygienist–administrator (health administrator, statistician, specialist in methods of instruction, specialist in sanitary education)		+	+
51 Doctor of general practice	+	+	+

Note: Specialists in gastroenterology, nephrology, haematology, neurosurgery, cardiovascular surgery, thoracic surgery, dental surgery (maxillary–facial surgery) can be appointed only to the in-patient sections of hospitals or to the consultative polyclinics of regional (territorial) and republican hospitals.

Source: Popov, *Problemi vrachebnikh kadrov*, pp. 55–6.

By about this time, it was recognized that the proliferation of specialties had become virtually uncontrolled. According to G. A. Popov in 1969 a total of 173 distinct specialist spheres had been designated in working units, despite the fact that only eighty-one separate posts were officially recognized. This situation was possible partly because of the absence of central control in this matter; there existed no standard practice which was binding on directors of health service organs and institutions. But in March 1970, after wide consultation, the USSR Ministry of Health grasped the nettle and issued the order: 'Concerning nomenclature of doctors' specialties and the nomenclature of doctors' posts in health service institutions'. As a result, the number of specialties was limited to fifty-one—the last being general practice.

The list of officially recognized specialties, which is given in Table 4.2, holds an interest both for what it contains and for what it leaves out. The differentiation within environmental health and oncology is especially striking and is without parallel in the list of specialties for England. The omission of geriatrics should also be mentioned since in England it now accounts for about as many hospital medical staff as does ENT. Further evidence of the priority assigned to health care for children is provided in the recognition of paediatric surgeon, paediatric ophthalmologist and specialist in the hygiene of children and adolescents. It should be added that the nomenclature of posts does not coincide fully with the list of specialties; some of the seventy-five posts are defined by reference to place of work or hierarchical position rather than technical content.

Turning now to the question of the territorial level at which various specialists may be employed, it can be remarked that even for a rural medical sector the permitted total is eight—including a general practitioner. At rural district level the number rises as high as forty-one. That these two sets of figures are far from being widely achieved can be regarded as less important than the strategy they embody and the prospect that they hold out for the future.

The Ministry's order of March 1970 required that a review of posts and specialties should be completed by the end of that year and forbade the establishment of posts which are not named in the official list. Incidentally, it also prohibited the creation of environmental health posts in curative units and of curative posts in environmental health units. The general effect of this reform has been clearly beneficial, according to G. A. Popov who played some part in bringing it about. 'The introduction of nomenclature for doctors' specialties', he wrote, 'has made possible fuller staffing of doctors' posts in the basic aspects of medical care—in general medicine, surgery, obstetrics and gynaecology, paediatrics, stomatology, and environmental health, especially in the ambulatory–polyclinic institutions.'[8]

The curbing of runaway specialization was closely related to a concern over imprecise usage of the term 'specialist'. In 1968, Popov had categorically stated that 'Most frequently the decision about which specialty this or that doctor should be assigned to is taken by the statistician when compiling the statistical return for an institution, being guided by the post occupied by the doctor and the field of his training'.[9] In other words, the obtaining of a recognized post-diploma qualification was not an essential prerequisite for practice as a specialist.

At that time, in fact, large numbers of specialists had undertaken no formal training course beyond their education in medical institute. In 1969 one writer commented that 'The greater proportion of young doctors used to commence work immediately as specialists in general medicine, another group from their first day in curative medicine became surgeons, ophthalmologists, otorhinolaryngologists and other specialists, without any preliminary specialization'. He went on to condemn that practice strongly, on the grounds that it 'has affected the quality of medical care given to the population, has led to the use of irrational methods of treatment and to increased duration of treatment which in turn has given rise to various economic costs for the community'.[10]

It is against the background of such criticism that one can set an announcement in a wide-ranging speech which was made to the Supreme Soviet by Health Minister Petrovski in June 1968. He stated that a scheme was to be introduced whereby intending doctors would be required to undertake 'primary specialization and practical training'. Experimental courses had proved successful and it had been decided to implement the reform throughout the whole country.

This decision obviously held major implications for the medical institutes—not only in respect of course content. According to the Minister, a serious constraint on raising the level of medical training was the 'antiquated material–technical base' at a number of establishments, including those for post-diploma courses. 'These institutions', he said, 'are frequently located in old buildings and not adequately supplied with up-to-date equipment.'[11] Although no figures have been obtained to prove the point, a sizeable increase in spending has undoubtedly occurred in this sector of the service during recent years.

The organizational changes entailed by the new system were completed first in faculties of curative medicine and paediatrics. Under the reformed curriculum, general medical education is completed within five years, to be followed by the *subordinatura* course during which students start to specialize. That is to say, students in faculties of curative medicine will become acquainted with one 'broad' specialty—general medicine or surgery or obstetrics and gynaecology. Students from paediatrics faculties have a choice between paediatrics, infectious diseases and children's surgery.

On successfully completing this sixth year, the student receives his diploma and proceeds to the internship (*internatura*) which lasts for one further year. During this time, young doctors may continue in their previous specialty or work in a 'narrow' specialty for which they have had suitable preparation. Thus an individual who has worked in general medicine for his *subordinatora* may proceed to an internship in, for example, neuropathology. Similarly a person who gained some knowledge of surgery in his sixth year can proceed to work in urology or traumatology or ophthalmology and so on. (But training in super-specialties such as haematology, endocrinology and nephrology is available only at a later stage.)[12] The *internatura* must be passed in a large hospital capable of providing supervision at an appropriate level of competence.

The general education in stomatology now lasts for $4\frac{1}{2}$ years and that in environmental health for $5\frac{1}{2}$ years.[13] Although arrangements for providing initial specialist training in these divisions of medicine differ in detail from the system described above, it appears that the same basic principle is being implemented.

It would be beyond the scope of this study to examine detailed consequences of the reform, such as the problems faced by local health service administrators in making suitable arrangements for the *internatura*. On the main issue, however, mention should be made of official satisfaction at the results as perceived so far. To give an example, as early as 1972, the USSR Minister of Health delivered the following summary verdict: 'Experience shows that the new system of training doctors affords a higher level of knowledge and practical skills'.[14]

It is by no means easy for a researcher to confirm the validity of that statement. But fragmentary support for it can be found in accounts of the activities of medical institutes written by members of their staff. An article relating to the Yaroslavl medical institute contains interesting data based on self-appraisal questions administered to young doctors; the authors were able to report that 'from year to year the number of unfavourable self-evaluations shows a decline'. In 1967–9, before the introduction of the *internatura*, thirty-six per cent of those completing the questionnaire considered that their practical experience in blood transfusion was unsatisfactory and fifty-seven per cent thought that their theoretical training and practice in reading electrocardiograms was clearly inadequate. Improvements followed the commencement in 1971 of internships at the curative institutions of Yaroslavl, Vologda and Kostroma

regions and of the Northern Railway. Some indication of the increase
in satisfaction among interns who had been students of the institute
is suggested by Table 4.3 which covers nine forms of activity in the
specialty of general medicine. It will be seen that the proportion of
respondents expressing dissatisfaction declined sharply in respect of
questions of fitness for work, electrocardiography and 'dispenserization'. The last-mentioned can be glossed as programmes for early
and periodic screening, diagnosis and treatment.

TABLE 4.3   *Doctors' dissatisfaction with training for various activities in general
medicine* (%)

Activity	Theoretical training			Practical training		
	1972	1974	1975	1972	1974	1975
Work in a polyclinic	34.0	35.0	35.0	33.3	35.7	32.8
Questions of fitness for work	18.5	5.6	4.8	19.3	10.9	5.1
Dispenserization	17.8	14.7	9.1	26.9	18.7	12.2
Emergency and first aid	8.0	23.2	8.3	44.0	12.7	15.5
Electrocardiography	34.8	9.5	8.0	44.0	13.0	17.3
Blood transfusion	4.0	6.0	6.6	43.5	19.0	29.2
Techniques of local anaesthetic	32.0	29.7	26.0	42.0	39.8	38.6
Delivery of infants	—	26.4	30.6	—	44.2	50.7
Practice of minor surgery	—	20.0	15.2	—	40.4	30.3

This study also provides evidence to suggest that the new form
of training is enhancing a pre-existing tendency towards compart-
mentalism in medical practice. Thus the authors write: 'It is established that during the internship a demarcation of professional
knowledge takes place in several types of universal medical activity,
for example delivery of infants and the practice of minor surgery'.
A closely connected point is that most of the young doctors who
subsequently failed to find satisfaction in their work were those who
had taken the *subordinatura* and *internatura* in one specialty but were
directed to work in another.[15]

RESEARCH TRAINING AND CONTINUING EDUCATION

Young doctors hoping to pursue academic careers in research and teaching can apply for entry to what is known as the *aspirantura*. This course, which normally lasts three years, is currently available at eighty medical institutes, twelve institutes for advanced medical training and 153 scientific research establishments. Entry is by competitive examination and there is now an emphasis on the need to increase the intake of specialists who already have publications to their name or have completed the two-year clinical *ordinatura*, a long-established type of specialist training in hospital. Supervised work for a research thesis is a cardinal feature of the *aspirantura*, successful completion of which results in a doctor receiving the degree of Candidate of Medical Science. Not all Candidates, however, are able to take up academic careers since the size of intakes is not closely related to the likely number of vacant posts. This situation was recently criticized in strong terms by *Meditsinskaya Gazeta* whose leader took the view that 'It is completely intolerable when, on completing the *aspirantura*, specialists are not given an opportunity for scientific work'. This unfortunate situation obtained in the Azerbaidzhan, Georgian, Kirgiz, Turkmen and Uzbek republics.[16]

Doctors who obtain permanent posts as researchers and teachers may subsequently submit more substantial theses based on their own research in order to qualify as a Doctor of Medical Science. That is the degree which confers the greatest prestige on a doctor; it is likely to assist—and reflect—success on a career ladder which gives access to far higher rewards, both tangible and intangible, than are available in ordinary practice. In or about 1976, health service research and teaching establishments contained 38,800 Candidates and 6,700 Doctors of Science.[17]

The new two-year training scheme described earlier was never intended to provide a once-for-all introduction to the requirements of work in a given specialty. Indeed the Minister followed up his announcement of it by stressing the significance of continuing education. 'Of course', he went on, 'a doctor will also continue to improve his qualifications throughout the whole course of his career.'[18] It should be added that a newly qualified doctor commits himself, when taking the professional oath, to the continuous improvement of his medical knowledge and skills.

The commitment of the state to post-diploma training has been manifested in recent years by the rapid increase in courses organized by institutes for advanced medical training and advanced training faculties at medical institutes. (There are now thirteen of the former and twenty-five of the latter.) According to one source, it is official policy that doctors practising in rural areas must take post-diploma courses every three years while those in towns should do so not less than once in five years.[19]

Despite an enormous expansion of training opportunities, however, it transpires that many specialists have not undertaken a course to update their knowledge and skills for some ten to fifteen years. Stomatologists and pharmacists are the least frequent attenders.

By 15 May each year, the republican health ministries should have submitted their plans for improving the qualifications of doctors—and pharmacists—to the Union Ministry's chief directorate of teaching establishments. The head of this department recently complained that only Latvia and Lithuania presented their submissions on time, while the RSFSR, Turkmen, Azerbaidzhan and Tadzhik republics were the worst offenders. He also deplored the fact that proposals frequently fail to be realistic. For example, in 1975 the Kazakh republic requested 4,624 passes of which only fifty-three per cent could be granted. But even the curtailed plan was shown to be excessive, since 169 of the passes were not taken up.[20]

The organization of these courses takes various forms, presumably in order to mitigate the difficulties facing doctors who wish to attend them. Disincentives must be especially powerful in the case of married women with children who would have to leave their homes in order to be in residence at the course centres; they may well prefer to follow the 'correspondence cycles' arranged by the institutes for advanced medical training. Study by correspondence must also recommend itself to directors of health service units since it obviates the need to arrange cover for temporarily absent staff.

It is not only the institutes that have formal responsibilities for the transmission of contemporary theory and practice in the various specialist fields. At a more local level, the larger hospitals contribute in a variety of ways, including correspondence and sandwich courses, towards the knowledge and skills of clinicians employed in their areas of influence. Specific mention can be made of the programmes which they arrange for staff of the sector and small district hospitals in rural areas. These programmes consist of practical training and independent reading during a period of some four months. Plans of study, incidentally, have been laid down in considerable detail by the USSR Ministry of Health; for example the 624-hour course in general medicine must include experience of nine specified 'diagnostic manipulations' and ten 'curative manipulations'.[21] This form of locally organized training appears to date back for some time and clearly represents one of the ways in which planners have sought to improve the quality of medical care available in remoter country areas.

Finally, brief mention should be made of the system of accreditation which is known as attestation. This came into existence in 1961 and the current regulations governing its operation are of less interest in this context than their general effect, which is to provide a measure of quality control and at the same time indicate the level of specialist competence attained by a given doctor as a result of post-diploma training and work experience. So far as the author is aware, only two levels of specialization have been defined. Certainly one text book states that during the years 1965 to 1969 a total of 66,200 doctors were confirmed in the first qualificatory category while over the same period 14,900 were assigned to a higher category.[22] It appears that additions to salary and improved job opportunities act as inducements to enter the first or advance into the second.

Attestation and the various types of post-diploma training are all entirely consistent with the theory—or dogma—of specialization as outlined at the start of this chapter. It is a matter for conjecture whether, in time to come, the health service bureaucrats will accept that fragmentation of medical practice has proceeded too far and will attempt to redress the balance. What does seem indubitable, however, is that Soviet orthodoxy will never be so revised as to endorse the validity of a single-entry, broad-gauged training for all intending doctors.

CHAPTER 5

Paramedical Personnel

More significant than doctors, in purely numerical terms, are the staff whom official sources refer to as intermediate medical personnel. In the Soviet Union, as elsewhere, these paramedical workers have an immense part to play in the fields of environmental health, prevention of illness and the treatment of patients. Predictably, their training is shorter and less academic than that of doctors and takes place in separate training establishments. As will be shown in this chapter, however, differentiation between Soviet doctors and paramedical staff is so far from being sharp and long-established that there are various significant forms of functional overlap between the two groups.

Numbers and Spatial Variation

It is appropriate first to refer to the rapid growth in the size of this aggregate group, which closely parallels the increase in doctors. As Table 5.1 shows, numbers rose more than threefold over the period 1950–74, from 719,400 to a massive 2,423,100. When these data are set against the total population of the USSR, it emerges that the ratio more than doubled, improving from 39.6 to 95.7 per 10,000 persons.

The ratio of paramedical staff to doctors is also an index to which health care planners pay some attention, on account of the importance attached to the maintenance of 'proportionality' between the two groups. It will be seen from the table that although this ratio improved from 2.71:1 in 1950 to 3.03:1 in 1974, a small decline

63

occurred after 1960. In other words, the increase in doctors since that time has been more rapid than the increase in paramedical staff. This trend is regarded as undesirable, to judge from a recently published textbook which firmly stated that 'it must be recognized that the most rational situation is for the growth rate of intermediate medical cadres to be slightly higher than that of doctors'.[1]

TABLE 5.1   *Number of intermediate medical personnel, 1950–1974*

| | End of years | | | |
	1950	1960	1970	1974
Absolute number	719,400	1,388,300	2,123,000	2,423,100
Personnel per 10,000 population	39.6	64.2	87.1	95.7
Personnel per doctor	2.71	3.22	3.18	3.03

Note: Intermediate medical personnel in the armed forces are excluded from the figures for 1950 and 1960 and are probably excluded from those for 1970 and 1974.

Sources: *Narodnoe Khozyaistvo SSSR* for 1970; and for 1974, *passim*.

By 1980, it is planned,[2] the numbers of paramedical workers will have risen to a total of 2,930,000. But this will yield a ratio of 3.06 staff per doctor, which is only a marginal improvement on the existing position. Perhaps the concept of proportionality is regarded as more strictly applicable to certain categories of staff than others. Certainly a leading article in *Meditsinskaya Gazeta*[3] singled out nurses and feldshers for special mention and stated that the ratio of these staff to doctors should move to a level of roughly 4:1. Whether that represents a firm policy objective on the part of the USSR Health Ministry was not made clear.

Of more direct practical relevance is the priority currently assigned in the health service, as in other sectors of the Soviet economy, to improving the training received by 'specialists with intermediate education'. In order to raise standards in medical and pharmaceutical schools (that is the Russian term), a range of measures are being introduced throughout the country. These include enlarging the schools and resiting them within the curtilage of major general hospitals and even of medical institutes. At a slightly less heroic level, a review of curricula has been undertaken for each type of training course. In a number of republics the management of the schools has been subject to a process of centralization.[4]

As is the case for doctors, the spatial distribution of paramedical workers reveals striking variation. This point is borne out by Table 5.2, which gives the numbers of staff-to-population ratios for the fifteen Union republics in 1950 and 1974. In the first of these two years, Azerbaidzhan was the best-supplied, with 46.9 staff per 10,000 persons, while Tadzhikistan came bottom of the league with only 21.9. Twenty-four years later, the Russian republic had moved up into first place but Tadzhikistan remained last. The range increased very substantially, from 25.0 to 42.5 staff per 10,000 persons.

TABLE 5.2 *Number of intermediate medical personnel by Union republic in 1950 and 1974*

Republic	End of 1950		End of 1974	
	Absolute number	Personnel per 10,000 population	Absolute number	Personnel per 10,000 population
RSFSR	450,500	43.8	1,362,500	101.9
Ukrainian SSR	136,400	36.6	470,500	96.4
Belorussian SSR	24,400	31.3	82,500	88.4
Uzbek SSR	15,100	23.2	101,100	73.9
Kazakh SSR	20,600	30.7	126,200	89.0
Georgian SSR	16,500	46.5	48,700	99.0
Azerbaidzhan SSR	13,800	46.9	44,700	79.8
Lithuanian SSR	5,800	22.6	29,300	89.0
Moldavian SSR	7,800	32.6	31,400	82.4
Latvian SSR	6,400	33.0	24,600	99.2
Kirgiz SSR	4,800	27.0	26,400	80.0
Tadzhik SSR	3,400	21.9	20,100	59.4
Armenian SSR	4,500	33.5	21,900	78.8
Turkmen SSR	5,400	43.8	19,000	76.0
Estonian SSR	4,000	35.7	14,200	99.2

Sources: *Narodnoe Khozyaistvo SSSR* for 1970. pp. 692–3; and for 1974. p. 730.

It is conceivable—though improbable—that those republics with a better endowment of paramedical workers have been consciously pursuing a policy of compensating for a shortage of doctors in their territory. If such a strategy had been successfully pursued, a negative association would be expected between the supply of these two main categories of health service cadres. In fact, however, a fairly high positive correlation can be shown to obtain between the doctor-to-population and paramedical staff-to-population ratios for the fifteen republics. In 1950 the value of the coefficient of correlation was 0.77 and it had risen to 0.84 by 1974. So in both years the republics which were under-doctored, according to the standards of the Union, also tended to be under-provided with paramedical workers, and this tendency became more marked over the period in question.

The requirements of individual republics are met, or very largely met, from the output of their own medical schools. These recently numbered over 650, of which 366 were located in the RSFSR and 115 in the Ukraine.[5] By the time of writing, the total may have been reduced due to the on-going process of enlargement and rationalization. As one might expect, not all types of training are necessarily provided under the same roof.

A SOVIET STRATEGY

Although republics with a relative shortage of doctors do not compensate by training above-average numbers of paramedical workers, nevertheless the concept of substitution can be said to apply in a different area—that of staffing practices. Over the years, many local health service agencies have found themselves unable to fill all the posts designated for doctors and, *faute de mieux*, have appointed intermediate medical personnel to these posts. By now, the practice is declining, although more rapidly in urban than in rural areas. It can be calculated that in 1970 in the main health service, 3.5 per cent of the occupied posts for doctors at urban units were filled by paramedical staff, while the figure for rural units was 5.8 per cent. By 1974 the corresponding figures had declined to 2.5 and 5.2 per cent.[6]

This practice would be seriously counter-productive in cases where a high degree of skill and training is essential to efficient functioning, but in towns it apparently operates mainly, if not solely, in respect of posts for general physicians and paediatricians appointed to serve an urban sector (*uchastok*). That is a territorial subdivision of the area served by a polyclinic and its size is such that one doctor can be assigned responsibility for the general oversight of the population resident in it. (More will be said on the subject in the next chapter.) Almost certainly, feldshers are the only type of paramedical staff eligible to act for doctors.

A survey which was undertaken in 1968 revealed that in towns feldshers occupied eight per cent (2,630) of posts designated for sector general physicians and 12.7 per cent (3,655) posts for sector paediatricians.[7] Given the increase in doctors and official disapproval of substitution, it is reasonable to assume that the situation has improved since that time. In the RSFSR, by 1976, sector doctors were being replaced by feldshers only in a limited number of regions in the Urals and western Siberia.[8]

The very fact that this practice has been reported and criticized by Soviet health bureaucrats points to an increasing emphasis on functional differentiation between the two main categories of medical cadres. But whether the trend has been accompanied by any appreciable widening of socio-occupational distance is most doubtful. It would certainly be quite erroneous to infer that the paramedical workers had suffered some form of defeat in a struggle with doctors who were seeking to enhance their status by means of restrictive practices. Indeed any consideration of the relationship between the various types of medical cadres must take into account the cardinal point that they have no opportunity to mount campaigns from separate power bases; in respect of corporate representation, all are embraced by a single union—the Union of Medical Workers. (On a point of detail, there exist various sections for different categories of staff.)

At a high level of generality this organization, like other unions, can be said to act primarily as an adjunct to the Communist Party and government of the USSR. But an important latent function specific to it is the inhibition of a sense of separate—and superior—identity among doctors. This point becomes clearer from a brief reference to the union's origins in the immediate post-revolutionary period. The crudely political role which it was created to play has been well described by Mark Field who traces in detail the way in which the Bolsheviks moved against those doctors' associations which were opposed to the new government. The paramedical workers' unions soon came under Bolshevik control and 'were encouraged, indeed urged, by the regime to assume leadership in medical affairs, to cut the physicians down to size, and to establish a central organ that would encompass *all* personnel in the medical or health field, regardless of specialization or education, an organization that would be receptive to the policies of the regime . . .' Just such a body, the Pan-Russian Union of Medical Workers, commenced its work in the spring of 1919 and soon membership of this organization became almost a precondition of employment in health service units. By the early 1930s, Field concludes, 'Little trace was left of the medical profession as an organized, self-governing, social group or social force'.[9]

It can be argued that in contemporary Soviet society, which attaches a high value to the possession of scientific and technological skills, the distinction between doctors and paramedical staff would have become more salient despite—the framework of a single union —were it not for another major constraining influence. This is the policy of enabling staff who have completed intermediate medical education and have practical experience of health care to acquire a doctor's diploma on, as it were, easy terms. That considerable numbers take advantage of this arrangement was shown by some of the findings in a survey of 15,000 doctors which was carried out in 1968 in four areas of the Russian republic. The percentage of all doctors who had formerly worked as paramedical staff was reported as 15.3 per cent; the figure for men being 17.8 per cent and that for women being rather lower at 15.4 per cent. As for length of time spent in their previous category, 27.2 per cent had served as paramedical workers for up to five years, fifty-seven per cent for between five and nine years while 15.8 per cent had served for ten years or more.[10]

Although a detailed account of this policy cannot be offered owing to lack of published information, it is important to give some indication of the lengths to which it has been carried in the post-war period. G. A. Popov states that in the academic year 1956/7 ten medical institutes in the Ukraine, drawing on experience from the early 1930s, inaugurated evening courses which enabled intermediate medical workers to qualify as doctors without any discontinuation of their current work. However, a degree of selection existed, in so far as entrance was limited to those who had completed paramedical training, had a record of at least three years' service, were under thirty-five and had passed the entrance examinations in those subjects which were also taught in courses held during the day. For the most part, the courses recruited staff from the towns in which the medical institutes were located. However, five of the Ukrainian institutes also accepted applicants 'from the periphery' who then transferred to vacant posts in the cities where they were to study.

By 1959 evening courses of that type existed in five of the Union republics and had 1,930 students. In 1961, the latest year for which Popov provides figures,[11] the number had risen to 3,870. Whether these and other non-traditional courses were judged to produce less than well-trained doctors remains unclear but certainly by the end of the 1960s a leading planner announced that medical (and pharmaceutical) institutes should provide only day-time courses for former paramedical staff. During the years 1971–5 all students were to be transferred to such courses, provided that the physical and technical resources of the institutes permitted.[12]

A question which naturally arises at this juncture is: what effect does the preferential transfer arrangement have on the calibre of paramedical workers and the quality of their work? A commonsense inference would be that the more strongly motivated and better-qualified are creamed off, as a result of which the ranks of nurses and feldshers in particular suffer a serious qualitative diminution. This is an inference for which the author has not found explicit confirmation in Soviet literature.

On a related theme, however, there is evidence to suggest that the health care planners, in their concern to facilitate entry to medical institute, have neglected the importance of career opportunities in retaining paramedical staff. This conclusion can be drawn from a letter by a feldsher working in Volgograd which was published in *Pravda* in 1975. His letter contains the following selected passages:

> It is no secret that that in hospitals and polyclinics there is some-times no one on duty. Without thinking twice, orderlies, nurses and feldshers collect their pay and change their occupation ... Compared to individuals who have completed a course in a technicum or paedagogical training school, medical workers of the intermediate level are at a considerable disadvantage. Their wages are lower, but their working conditions are no easier. For example, the feldshers of sanitary–epidemiological stations spend half their time investigating working conditions in industrial enter-prises. They have to take samples of air in hot workshops and places where there is a lot of dust and gas. But they are not provided with special clothing and footwear ... Technicians of almost all types and primary school teachers can improve their

qualifications at correspondence and evening faculties of appropriate higher educational institutes. But we do not have such an opportunity ... The turnover among feldshers, midwives and nurses makes it difficult to care for patients. It seems that health service organs should show more concern for medical personnel. Then there won't be notices which read 'Wanted for permanent employment' hanging in hospitals and polyclinics.[13]

Referring back to the feldsher's complaint about opportunities for obtaining additional qualifications, it should be added that, in fact, two main types of post-diploma courses exist for paramedical staff—specialization and further training. However, a survey published in 1975 discovered that only 14.8 per cent of staff in Moscow had undertaken specialization while a mere 2.2 per cent had followed further training courses.[14] The author of the survey did not speculate about the reasons for these low figures or about their bearing on the quality of work undertaken by the various categories of staff.

THE ROLE OF THE RURAL FELDSHER

At this point it is appropriate to examine the relative size of the categories or specialties (to use Russian terminology) which make up the broad grouping of paramedical workers. In the statistical yearbooks, ten specialties are listed and a residual group of some size is easily discovered. Table 5.3 records the breakdown of staff in the years 1950 and 1974.

Predictably enough, nurses substantially outnumber the other specialties, representing 45.2 per cent and 48.9 per cent of the total in the two years in question. The next largest group, by far, consists of feldshers, who accounted for 22.2 per cent of all staff in 1950 and 21.7 per cent in 1974. It seems certain that this group embraces not only feldshers but also feldsher–sanitarians whose training, as their name indicates, is oriented towards environmental health. But separate record is made of the hybrid feldsher–midwives who declined from 5.8 to 3.2 per cent of all paramedical workers.

Although many feldshers work in urban areas under the direct supervision of doctors, they should be seen as significant mainly for the independent role they play in the rural health service. Especially in remoter areas, vividly described by the Russians as bears' corners, they have been indispensable as doctor–surrogates since Tsarist times. As late as the 1970s, sections of their curriculum at training school were still predicated on the assumption that they would continue to perform important clinical functions on an unsupervised basis. Of the course which covered general medicine the USSR Health Ministry wrote:

> This course is intended to train the feldsher to give the patient medical care in the absence of the physician, correctly and without supervision. He is also taught to prescribe an appropriate treatment, to carry out basic medical procedures, to organize and attend to the care of the sick, to prepare case reports for visits to a physician ...[15]

TABLE 5.3 *Intermediate medical personnel by specialty in 1950 and 1974*

Specialty	End of 1950		End of 1974	
	Number	*%*	*Number*	*%*
Feldshers	160,000	22.2	525,100	21.7
Feldsher–midwives	42,000	5.8	78,500	3.2
Midwives	66,500	9.2	244,100	10.1
Assistants to environmental health doctors and assistants to epidemiologists	18,500	2.6	45,500	1.9
Nurses	325,000	45.2	1,185,500	48.9
Medical laboratory assistants	25,300	3.5	105,300	4.3
x-ray technicians and x-ray laboratory assistants	7,500	1.0	29,800	1.2
Dental technicians	6,700	0.9	30,000	1.2
Disinfestors* and disinfectionists	27,000	3.8	87,000	3.6
Residual group†	40,900	5.7	92,300	3.8
TOTALS	719,400	100	2,423,100	100

* This is a conjectural translation of *dezinstruktori*.
† Not given in source; obtained by subtracting numbers listed under each specialty from the grand total.

Sources: *Narodnoe Khozyaistvo SSSR* for 1970, p. 692; and for 1974, p. 730.

The feldsher's independance is at a maximum in the peripheral units of a rural medical sector known as feldsher and feldsher–midwife points. (The latter term conventionally extends to the former as well.) These buildings are located not only in outlying villages but also at the sites of rural industrial concerns, such as timber works, and on state and collective farms; the cost of their construction is frequently met by the enterprises whose work force they serve. Their activities are performed under the general direction of doctors of the rural sector hospital or district-centre hospital, if one is situated in the sector, and their work schedule forms an integral part of the scheme for the whole sector. It is evident that the quality of this direction from a superordinate unit will inevitably be subject to variation. The textbook on which this section draws cautiously spells out a crucial proviso when it states: 'If the sector doctor carries out his task systematically and supervises the fulfilment of his recommendations, then as a rule in such a medical sector the feldsher–midwife points function well, display initiative and achieve all the objectives set before them'.

Notwithstanding the development of rural medical units staffed by fully trained doctors, a vast expansion in the network of feldsher–midwife points has occurred during the last decade or so. By 1972 the total for the USSR stood at 89,718, which makes them by far the most numerous of health service units. It can be noted in passing that the figure includes some mobile points such as those used in the Kazakh republic to provide curative and prophylactic care for the shepherds who lead a nomadic existence with their flocks. Mention can also be made of the fact that in many areas the services of a feldsher are available in the fields during times of peak activity such as harvest.

In recent years, variations on the basic organizational form have been devised which considerably extend the scope of this unit. For example, the Moldavian republic has introduced what is known as a rural health post (on what scale is not clear) which brings together under one roof feldsher–midwife point, milk kitchen, pharmacy point and collective-farm maternity home. In addition, this multi-purpose building will occasionally include the prophylactorium, a form of sanatorium, owned by a collective farm. In the Tsimlinsk district of Rostov region from 1969 onwards, nine so-called zonal base points have been established to serve sectors with a population of 3,000 to 3,500. As well as having a wider range of full-time staff than usual, these points are the venue for out-patient clinics held by visiting specialist doctors.

From time to time in the development of feldsher–midwife points, enthusiasm has outrun the dictates of rational planning. Partly to prevent wasteful excesses, in 1966 the Union Health Ministry issued an order which laid down separate staffing norms for units of different sizes serving populations ranging from 700 to 3,000. Four categories of staff are involved: feldsher, midwife, community nurse (*patronazhnaya sestra*) and orderly, but only for the feldsher is there a full-time post in every case. It is important to note that the order was not intended to be applied inflexibly; health ministries of the Union republics have the right to introduce additional posts in individual cases and the population norms are also subject to qualification. Thus villages containing 300–700 persons may acquire a point if they are located at a distance of more than five kilometres from any health service unit. And although the establishment of two points in a single village is normally forbidden, permission may be granted by the local health service organs in cases where the population amounts to 3,000 and the points are three to four kilometres apart.

In 1973 the Union Health Ministry issued another order whose main importance appears to reside in its specification of functions to be performed by the feldsher–midwife points. These include the following:

1   Execution of measures directed to:
    (a) Prophylaxis and the reduction of morbidity including infectious diseases; prophylaxis and reduction of morbidity from parasitic and occupational diseases, accidents and food poisoning among collective farmers, the workers on state farms and other enterprises;
    (b) The reduction of mortality including infant and maternal mortality;
    (c) Raising the levels of sanitary-hygienic culture among the population.

2   Providing the population with initial medical care.

3   Participating in on-going sanitary inspection of establishments for children and adolescents, communal, food, industrial and other premises, and of the water supply and waste disposal in populated areas.

4   Carrying out home visits for indicators of epidemics with the object of discovering infected patients, persons who have been in contact with them and persons suspected of being carriers of infectious diseases.

5   Notifying the local sanitary–epidemiological station in the approved manner about infections, parasitic and occupational diseases, food poisoning in the population and infringements of the regulations concerning sanitation and hygiene.[16]

In its preoccupation with preventive medicine and environmental health activities, this order probably reflects a shift in official thinking about the place of the feldsher in rural medical care. A few years later, a deputy Health Minister of the USSR certainly revealed the existence of a new policy when he said that further expansion of the network of feldsher–midwife points must not occur and that an increase in the volume of out-patient treatment provided by paramedical staff in rural areas must not be permitted. He went on to state that the activity of feldsher–midwife points should be more widely and more purposefully concentrated on the provision of prophylactic measures and that this type of unit ought to be more firmly involved in dispenserization and the rehabilitation of patients.[17]

TABLE 5.4   *Out-patient care provided for the rural population in 1970 and 1975*

	1970	1975
Number of visits to doctors*	353,620,500	425,323,200
Average visits per person	3.4	4.3
Number of visits to feldshers and other paramedical staff	415,937,300	436,699,500
Average visits per person	4.0†	4.4

* Includes visits by rural population to urban units.
† Excludes the Moldavian SSR.

Source: *Sovetskoe Zdravookhranenie*, 1, 1977, p. 20.

That a massive and, indeed, increasing amount of medical care was being provided by feldshers and other paramedical staff is shown by Table 5.4, which relates to the whole Union. In 1970 the average number of visits to these staff stood at 4.0 per rural inhabitant and had grown to 4.4 by 1975. The latter figure was slightly higher, it must be insisted, than the rate of consultations with doctors, although that had risen sharply over the period in question.

The sheer volume of first-line care which feldshers provide makes all the more serious a variety of shortcomings in their diagnostic competence and methods of treatment. By the mid-1960s, attention was being focussed on this major problem and a study summarized in *Meditsinskaya Gazeta* in that year contained some most disquieting findings. It related to three districts in the Belorussian republic with a total population of around 130,000 of whom 75.4 per cent lived in areas served by feldsher–midwife points. During one year, 52.2 per cent of visits to health care units were made to doctors and 41.9 per cent to feldshers. The researchers discovered that feldshers had special difficulties in recognizing diphtheria, dysentery and tuberculosis and also made mistakes in diagnosing diseases of the cardiovascular system. In cases of serious illness, when the feldsher has established a diagnosis and given essential preliminary treatment, he is obliged to refer the patient to a specialist; the survey found that this rule was frequently disregarded. As for bone fractures, doctors saw 107 out of a total recorded number of 217 cases. Similarly only 484 cases of focal pneumonia reached a doctor out of a recorded total of 1,573 cases. The corresponding figures for diphtheria were seven out of thirteen and for dysentery twenty out of thirty-five. The numbers of patients attending hospital for observation were also below what could have been predicted. Out of 252 persons suffering from appendicitis according to the feldsher's diagnosis, only eighty in fact went to hospital and out of six recorded as suffering from intestinal obstruction only one attended.[18]

There can be little doubt that for certain health service planners such research findings contained a most significant policy implication: that the clinical functions of feldshers should be reallocated to doctors. Probably the first republic to take action along these lines was Georgia, which started with the advantages, as may be recalled, of a relatively high population density and an especially favourable doctor-to-patient ratio. As early as 1967, the Health Minister of Georgia stated quite categorically: 'We consider that the rural population should visit only a doctor for initial medical care'. He went on to describe how new ambulatories (clinics) staffed by doctors had been opened to serve areas within a radius of three to four kilometres, making possible the closure of many units staffed by paramedicals: feldsher–midwife points, small sector hospitals and maternity homes at collective farms. As a result, the proportion of patients who received initial care from doctors had risen to about eighty per cent.[19]

More recently, the Ukraine adopted a similar strategy and has made considerable progress towards ensuring that the whole countryside is served by medically staffed ambulatories. From the Lvov region, for example, it is reported that during the years 1970–73 the number of visits to ambulatories rose from 1.6 to 3.2 per rural inhabitant while attendances at feldsher–midwife points fell from 2.9 to 2.1 per person.[20] To what extent other republics have followed suit is unclear.

In the longer term, according to current orthodoxy, the provision of initial medical attention by feldshers will be restricted to emergency treatment. However, it is clear that progress in achieving this objective is bound to be far slower in some parts of the USSR than in others, due to the great variation in factors such as density of population, average size of villages, ease of communications and climatic conditions, let alone the problem of retaining doctors in the backwoods. In some areas, apparently, something of an interim strategy has been adopted which entails improving the feldsher's clinical competence by various means such as refresher courses, training in elementary laboratory techniques and more effective oversight by doctors. So large numbers of feldshers will almost certainly continue in practice as doctor-surrogates for several decades to come.

CHAPTER 6

Out-patient Services

By way of introduction, it should be explained that the title of this chapter is not intended to convey only the limited associations which attach to the term out-patient as used in the British health service. The topic under discussion is in fact the totality of care provided by doctors for patients other than those occupying beds in hospitals and comparable institutions. In Russian parlance this is the ambulatory–polyclinical service, a clumsy phrase for which it seemed desirable to substitute the alternative chosen.

Out-patient services, as defined above, are organized in a range of institutional settings among which the most important and best-known in the West is the polyclinic. This type of unit predates the Revolution and was constructed at public expense on an increasing scale from the 1880s onwards. As the name implies, a polyclinic caters for a variety of presenting symptoms and it can be differentiated on that score from units which offer treatment only in a single specialty.

According to the statistical yearbook, the total number of institutions providing out-patient care in 1950 was 36,200; the figure for 1974 was 35,900. This decline, which results from a process of re-organization and enlargement over a number of years, certainly does not imply any reduction in the volume of care received by the population. Basic indicators of activity in this sector of the service are the total number of consultations with doctors, whether in institutions or at home, and the average number of consultations per person. The consultation rate in urban areas has actually risen quite substantially since 1960, from an average of 8.5 contacts per person to 11.1 in 1974.

This index varies considerably between republics. Thus in 1974 it stood at 8.9 per person in the towns of the Turkmen republic but was as high as 13.5 in Latvia. For large manufacturing towns such as Moscow, Leningrad, Baku, Kiev, Odessa, Kharkov, Kramatorsk, Voroshilovgrad and Donetsk, out-patient consultations amount to some 12–15 per inhabitant each year. In rural areas contacts with the doctor are at a much lower level; as was recorded in the previous chapter, the all-Union figure was 4.0 per rural inhabitant in 1974. In Azerbaidzhan and Tadzhikistan, the rural consultation rate was only 2.7 per person but the Baltic republics, not surprisingly, had a more impressive record and the figure for Lithuania was as high as 5.7 per person.

TABLE 6.1   *Out-patient consultations in 1974*

	Urban population		Rural population	
	Number (000s)	Consultations per person	Number (000s)	Consultations per person
Total consultations with a doctor	1,683,425.2	11.12	406,902.5	4.04
Consultations at:				
polyclinics, ambulatories, consultation centres and dispensaries	1,501,426.7	9.92	390,281.7	3.88
home	119,248.6	0.79	10,498.9	0.10
emergency service	62,749.9	0.41	4,742.8	0.05
sanitary aviation service			1,379.1	0.01
Consultations with intermediate medical personnel	483,428.3	3.20	417,255.9	4.14

Source: Popov, *Ekonomika i planirovanie zdravookhraneniya*, p. 159.

By no means all consultations were for purposes of diagnosis and treatment. In 1972 in the main health service, 66.6 per cent of all visits to a doctor by the urban and rural population were recorded as being in connection with illness or dispenserization, while 33.4 per cent were for health checks. Since a degree of compulsion operates in the case of the latter, it would be stretching a point to suggest that these contacts with a doctor were initiated by the patient.[1]

As may be seen from Table 6.1, which relates to 1974, the vast majority of consultations occur in polyclinics, ambulatories, consultation centres and dispensaries. (Apparently no breakdown of figures as between these different types of units is published for the Union as a whole.) It is interesting that home visiting, much of which is to children, accounted for only 7.08 per cent and 2.58 per cent of all contacts with a doctor in urban and rural areas respectively. Out-patient activity by the organizationally distinct emergency service represented 3.7 per cent of contacts in towns and 1.2 per cent in rural areas. The vital function of the sanitary air service in providing access to a doctor is obviously out of all proportion greater than the number of consultations recorded for it. The importance of para-medical staff as providers of initial medical care in the countryside was referred to in the last chapter and the table shows that average contacts with these personnel are not so much lower in urban areas.

THE POLICY OF UNIFICATION

A striking feature of many units providing treatment for the ambulant is that they are located within the same set of buildings as a hospital. Moreover, even when they are not located within the same curtilage, many out-patient units are still administered as an integral part of a neighbouring hospital. In this respect the Soviet Union contrasts very sharply with the United Kingdom where the delivery of medical care from general practitioners' surgeries or health centres is geographically and administratively dissociated from hospitals.

It was in 1947 that the USSR Ministry of Health instigated a reorganization of major dimensions by deciding to 'unify' most hospitals and out-patient units in urban areas. The main objectives of this policy included bringing together successive stages of treatment, introducing the medical 'culture' of hospitals into polyclinics, broadening the experience of hospital doctors, raising doctors' qualifications and improving the quality of service rendered to the population.[2] Presumably the last-mentioned should be seen as the basic goal for which the others were instrumental so far as they represent essential preconditions.

The policy of unification was implemented uniformly throughout the USSR within a comparatively short period of time. By 1951, in

wns, ninety-nine per cent of general hospitals and eighty-nine
 ent of children's hospitals (non-infectious) had been unified with
out-patient units, and the number of independent polyclinics, etc.,
had dropped by seventy-five per cent.[3] Key management features
of the unified establishments were: a single chief doctor, one budget
and one set of established posts for doctors, paramedical staff and
so on.

But within a short time it became clear that the shot-gun marriage
was operating very much to the detriment of out-patient care. This
result flowed primarily from the recommended arrangements for
manpower deployment; one of these entailed shift work in three
separate areas of activity—on the wards, in the polyclinic and out
in the district. A variant on this 'three-link' system was the 'two-
link', under which the total work load was divided between duties
in hospital and polyclinic together with district. For various reasons,
not all of which are clear, this system created a gross imbalance in
the man-hours actually available to the hospital on the one hand
and the out-patient service on the other. According to an authoritative survey carried out in 1952, the time available for consultation
in general medical departments of polyclinics had declined by 36.2
per cent following unification, whereas the time available for the
same speciality in hospitals had increased by 99.7 per cent. A reduction occurred in the quality of out-patient practice—consultations
had to be more hurried—and a decrease was registered in the volume
of out-patient work, more particularly in the field of preventive
measures.

It is interesting that, in abreaction to the arrangements recommended by the USSR Ministry of Health, a number of areas fairly soon
adopted the system of 'alternation'. Under it one group of doctors
would work full-time in the polyclinic and another in the hospital,
with a change-over every few months. This cyclical system, which
ensured a more predictable supply of manpower for the out-patient
service, was endorsed—and the three-link system condemned as unsuitable—by a Ministry order issued in April 1954. It was revealingly
entitled: 'Concerning measures for the further improvement of
organizational forms of medical service for the population and the
correction of mistakes committed in the unification of hospitals and
polyclinic establishments'. Apparently the system of alternation still
operates in united establishments, although it may have been

modified in detail as functional differentiation has assumed greater importance than interchangeability of staff.

A feature which arose from the policy of unification—and served to entrench it—was the large-scale construction of new hospitals and polyclinics on the same or neighbouring sites. The spatial relationship of existing premises was also affected by the process of upgrading and expanding more suitable accommodation, accompanied as it was by the closure of small units which had become surplus to requirements. In the Russian Republic in 1952, only 54.7 per cent of establishments under a single administration had ward blocks and polyclinic on a single site or within a distance of one kilometre. By 1959, however, the figure had risen to 70.5 per cent.[4]

Throughout the 1950s, the more undesirable consequences of unification continued to be perceived and dissatisfaction voiced. In January 1960 an all-Union conference on the polyclinic service created an opportunity for medical administrators to focus attention on the problems and formulate new policies. At this conference 'unanimous approval' greeted a demand for the establishment of separate financing for hospitals and polyclinics and for a more rational allocation of cadres as between wards and the polyclinic. Moreover, it was resolved that future building plans should provide for independent polyclinics in addition to those sited at hospitals.[5] Emphasis was also laid on the more general objectives of extending the scope of out-patient care and improving its quality.

After 1960 a fairly rapid growth occurred in the number of non-unified polyclinics serving the urban population. Between 1960 and 1968 they rose by 47.2 per cent while unified establishments increased by 14.7 per cent. Nevertheless, non-united ambulatories and polyclinics in urban areas still numbered only 2,041 in 1968 as against the 9,457 united establishments.[6] It is interesting to note that the size of the two types of polyclinic differed little in respect of established posts for doctors. Thus in 1969 the non-unified units had an average of 29.5 while the unified variant had 28.0 posts. Polyclinic departments attached to rural district hospitals had considerably smaller establishments—an average of 17.0 posts for doctors. Going on to other types of unit, dispensaries had 13.0 posts in towns and 6.0 posts in rural areas while rural ambulatories unattached to hospitals had 2.0 posts.[7]

The position reached by 1970 is indicated in Table 6.2 which refers to both urban and rural areas. From the figures given there it can be calculated that seventy-five per cent of all units were administratively unified with various types of institution containing in-patient accommodation. A substantially higher percentage could probably be obtained if there were no separate entry for health points staffed by a doctor. It seems highly probable that, as an entire category, these small and unsophisticated units form outposts, so to speak, of polyclinics serving industrial enterprises or district polyclinics and therefore should be regarded in this context as being 'united' with them.

TABLE 6.2   *Out-patient units staffed by doctors in 1970 (main health service)*

	Number of units
Units forming part of:	
Regional hospitals	198
Town hospitals	4,658
Rural district hospitals in urban settlements	2,567
Rural district hospitals in rural areas	1,469
Rural sector hospitals	11,325
Children's hospitals (for non-infectious diseases)	1,024
Maternity homes	695
Dispensaries	3,737
Other types of hospital	526
Non-unified out-patient units*	4,763
Health points staffed by doctors	3,268
Self-standing dental surgeries	783
TOTAL	35,013

* Includes units for children and for women and units situated at health resorts.

Source: *Sovetskoe Zdravookhranenie*, 2, 1972, p. 86.

In 1969 a precise indication of government policy concerning the construction of polyclinics was given by a leading planner when writing about health service development envisaged under the ninth five-year plan. Dr V. V. Golovteev stated that 'The most expedient structural form for a curative–prophylactic establishment capable of providing all forms of out-patient and in-patient care to a population remains, as before, the polyclinic united with a hospital'. This denotes not merely administrative unification but the conlocation of the two divisions on a single site. However, this model was to apply in towns where an approximate correspondence obtained between wards and out-patient unit in respect of specified factors: volume of work, numbers of patients served and location. Golovteev went on to say that in large towns where the building of hospitals with 600 or more beds was intended, it was permissible to create a network of independent polyclinics and also branch polyclinics in distant districts and in industrial enterprises.

At this time there also emerged an interesting new policy which entailed designating certain polyclinics as consultative centres. It became a requirement that in towns with 150–200,000 inhabitants there should be polyclinics which, in consort with the relevant in-patient departments, should provide a service for the whole town or district in respect of narrow specialities such as endocrinology, urology, cardiorheumatology, gastroenterology and so on.[8] In this way the increasing specialization of medicine fostered the partial emergence of what might be termed a two-tier system of polyclinics.

The additional attention being devoted to out-patient provision at this time is also reflected in the fact that the national economic plan included a target figure for the construction of polyclinics and similar buildings. The figure denotes not the number of units but their total workload expressed in terms of visits per shift. At the end of the ninth five-year plan, Golovteev reported that in place of projected additional building to cater for 402,000 consultations per shift, the increased capacity could cater for over 560,000 consultations. He also reported that an increase had occurred in the number of large new polyclinics of standard design capable of handling 750–1,200 patients per shift, while existing buildings had been enlarged and fitted with modern equipment.[9]

The reliance on large polyclinics necessarily entails some degree of centralization and concentration of services, the advantages of which are not always appreciated by patients who have to undertake long or difficult journeys. And the fact that the problem of location recently figured in a magazine article suggests that planners are beginning to recognize the validity of consumer opinion in this matter—even if no major change of policy is likely to result. The article included the following discussion:

> If you can reach a polyclinic on foot in five minutes, well and good. But what if it takes twenty minutes, thirty or even more?

What if you have to travel by tram or trolleybus and transfer to another line? In that case getting to the polyclinic (most commonly visited by persons who are not in good health) may be harder than sitting in the queue waiting at the polyclinic and may do a person more harm than poorly administered treatment.

It would seem simple enough to replace each large polyclinic with several smaller ones. Patients often make this suggestion when they fill out questionnaires. But let us assume that we did that. The gratified inhabitant of a sector would come to the polyclinic closest to his home, only to be sent to another, central one where he could find the specialized treatment he needed, a room supplied with complicated and expensive equipment of a kind that could not be supplied to each of the small polyclinics envisaged (where such equipment would most probably not be needed much of the time). The same would be true of specialists, whose role has steadily grown with the development of medical science ...

Evidently large polyclinics are necessary, but how can they serve those who live far away? For example, what about the mother who must take a crowded bus with her two small children to reach a children's consultation centre?

It is not easy to find the best solution ...[10]

FRAGMENTED CARE

As would be expected, the out-patient units for specific population groups or disease categories are staffed largely or entirely by specialists in the appropriate field. But it is a key feature of polyclinics for adults that they too are organized essentially along the lines of specialist departments—in keeping with the general strategy of specialization in medical practice which was discussed in chapter 4. Moreover, so far as the author has been able to ascertain, patients have an opportunity to refer themselves to the basic specialists. Thus someone with an eye complaint can proceed directly to the ophthalmologist and a patient suffering from earache can go to the ENT department. (Although some form of initial sorting process may operate at the registration point, this will not necessarily inhibit self-referral.) The extent to which the specialists act as consultants seeing patients referred to them by other doctors working in their polyclinic—or elsewhere—will vary with the department concerned.

It is certainly the case that one specialty, general medicine,

TABLE 6.3   *Consultation rates per person in 1970 (main health service)*

Specialty	Urban population	Rural population
General medicine	3.05	1.03
Cardiorheumatology	0.08	0.01
Endocrinology	0.07	0.02
Infectious diseases	0.09	0.02
Physiotherapy	0.11	—
Surgery	0.84	0.32
Traumatology and orthopaedics	0.18	0.02
Urology	0.06	0.01
Oncology	0.07	0.04
Obstetrics and gynaecology	0.71	0.21
Tuberculosis	0.25	0.14
Neuropathology	0.37	0.10
Psychiatry	0.11	0.04
Ophthalmology	0.56	0.16
Otorhinolaryngology	0.61	0.14
Dermato-venereology	0.56	0.15
Curative physical culture and supervision of persons undertaking physical culture and sport	0.07	—
Paediatrics	1.52	0.41
Stomatology	1.29	0.58
TOTAL	10.6	3.4

Note: These data include home visits.

Source: Popov, *Problemi vrachebnikh kadrov*, p. 100.

overshadows all others in respect of out-patient consultations. Even so, in 1970 it accounted for only 3.05 contacts per urban inhabitant out of a total of 10.6 and only 1.03 per rural inhabitant out of a total of 3.4. As can be seen from Table 6.3, the three next largest workloads were carried by paediatrics, stomatology and surgery. In a separate breakdown for home vists, general medicine would occupy a far more prominent position but that is because such activity figures prominently in the job specification of sector general physicians.

Over the years, the organization of out-patient care in polyclinics has developed along increasingly fragmented lines as new posts have been established in narrow specialties and more sophisticated equipment is provided for the appropriate consulting rooms. Staffing norms for the various specialties have been laid down by the USSR

Ministry of Health and the most recent, so far as urban polyclinics are concerned, were published in 1968. However, it is relevant to range back to an order issued by the USSR Health Ministry in July 1960 which required, among other things:

(a) the establishment of one post in urology and one in endocrinology per 50,000 urban population;

(b) the organization at one of the polyclinics in regional and large manufacturing centres of a special consultative clinic in orthopaedics for adults and children;

(c) the organization of a round-the-clock traumatology service in polyclinics of towns with a population of over 200,000.

By 1968 a considerable increase in capacity had taken place in the areas of specialist practice singled out for executive action. For example, in that year there were 2,078 endocrinology rooms in polyclinics—nine times the figure for 1959. A rapid growth also occurred in the number of rooms for cardiorheumatology, a sub-specialty of general medicine which the Ministry wished to see develop. That development casts revealing light on patterns of morbidity in the USSR, as also does the increase in rooms for the treatment of infectious diseases.[11] It is worth adding that the staffing norms of 1968 recommended one post in cardiorheumatology and one in infectious diseases for every 50,000 adults in urban areas.[12]

At this point brief reference can also be made to the development of specialization in the work of the emergency service, which deals with sudden illness, serious accidents, out-of-hours requests for home visits and the like. In towns and large rural districts, so-called brigades have been organized in a number of fields including cardiology, reanimation, neurology, toxicology, paediatrics and intensive care. With their specially equipped transport, these flying squads form a dramatic element in the Soviet health service and have received favourable publicity in the West. But whether this innovation has met with full acceptance is not clear; Popov cautiously notes that an in-depth study of their effectiveness is still awaited.[13]

For the deployment of an out-patient specialist's time official guidelines have been issued which specify how many patients per hour should be seen at home and how many in the polyclinic. Rather than list these norms, however, it seems more useful to refer to a time-study carried out (probably during the mid-1960s) at polyclinics in Rostov-on-Don, Benderi, Orel and Kishinev. This showed that the average time spent per consultation was significantly lower than the norm in certain specialties. Thus paediatricians spent 7.4 minutes, obstetrician-gynaecologists 8.8 minutes and neuropathologists nine minutes, as opposed to the intended twelve in each case.

From those figures it could still be concluded that each patient enjoys an opportunity to discuss his or her case at some length and receives a very full examination from a clinician who is not pressed for time. But the figures tell a somewhat different story when broken down by the various activities which a doctor performs. The average time spent by a general physician on questioning a patient was 2.4 minutes, while giving advice and conducting an examination took 1.8 and 2.9 minutes respectively. A further 4.5 minutes per consultation were required for the completion of medical documents.[14] Although the source is silent on this point, it seems likely that the sizeable amount of time spent on documentation can be explained largely by the need to issue patients with certificates of various kinds, rather than by the copious recording of case notes.

These figures by themselves are obviously of less interest than the patient's overall impression of what they entail for him, and that impression, on the evidence, is somewhat critical. The article quoted earlier in connection with the difficulty of travelling to large polyclinics also conveys a vivid picture of disappointed expectations and minimal interaction between doctor and patient. It includes the passage:

> Now let us assume that your child has fallen ill and you have called a paediatrician to your home. You would like to describe to the doctor in detail how the illness developed, tell him that something of the sort happened once before, that there were some medicines that the child took willingly and others he flatly refused to take. Your doorbell rings. The doctor comes in quite out of breath and after a brief greeting makes for the telephone: 'Zina, it is I. Have I had any more calls? Let me write them down. No, I still have three more home visits to make and may be delayed'. The detailed account you mean to give the doctor freezes on your lips. However, he would not have listened to it in any case. Once he has examined the child, filled out a sick-leave certificate [for the mother] and written the prescription, he dashes on to his next call.

Numerous studies have established the enormous importance of the doctor's behaviour, the psychotherapeutic effect of a friendly talk with the patient. The doctor should not only know the patient's ailment but his frame of mind as well. But can we hope for any elementary attentiveness at all if, according to the figures of one of the studies, we spend only five to eight minutes in the doctor's room and if only half or a third of that time is given to the examination itself and to discussion, the remainder being used to fill out certificates? That is why sociological research has established that the public is constantly dissatisfied with the lack of attentiveness on the part of doctors.[15]

URBAN SECTORS AND THEIR DOCTORS

The foregoing criticism acquires enhanced significance when set against ideal-type descriptions of the sector principle which entails a single doctor carrying a general responsibility for the population resident in one subdivision (sector) of the area served by his polyclinic. From some of the glossier statements it might be supposed that the Soviet Union has somehow recreated key elements of the British general practitioner service, and Soviet terminology in fact includes the phrase 'family doctor'. However, the attempt to institutionalize a generalist service encounters a basic difficulty: it runs counter to the main thrust of Soviet medicine and the intellectual presuppositions which underlie specialization.

Even the sector principle itself has had to be modified in order to take account of the fragmentation of first-line care. Thus there can be no one type of sector doctor: adults are served by staff of the general medicine department while children are the responsibility of paediatricians. Sectors also exist in the field of obstetrics and gynaecology and tuberculosis, though these do not figure at all prominently in the literature. The concept of family doctoring seems even less applicable when it is appreciated that the practice areas of general physicians and paediatricians are not necessarily coterminous. In the late 1940s and early 1950s, official policy favoured the so-called single sector but in 1960, on account of the problems that had arisen, the Union Health Ministry decided to permit the creation of paediatric sectors by reference to child population data alone.

Over the years, frequent mention has been made of the increase in the number of urban sectors, a development to which much importance has been attached, at least since 1956. The significance of this *terminus a quo* is that the Union Health Ministry then propounded the view that 'for the further reduction of morbidity and mortality it was necessary above all to break down the medical sectors into smaller units'. Between the years 1955 and 1968, general medical sectors increased in number from 17,114 to 31,949 and their paediatric equivalents from 15,397 to 33,153. While some part of the increase is to be explained by reference to urban population growth, much of it reflects the progressive lowering of the average number of persons per sector.[16]

The standard establishment figures for urban polyclinics, issued in 1968, include five posts for sector general physicians per 10,000 adult population. Put in another way, this represents one post per 2,000 persons. In 1974, however, there was only one post for every 2,832 persons, which is well below the desired figure.[17] Posts for sector doctors prove more difficult to fill than those for other specialties and, as was shown earlier, the employment of paramedical staff as substitutes is resorted to, though to a decreasing extent.

The comparative unpopularity of this type of work can also be inferred from a high turn-over rate of staff. A survey published in 1975, which related to Moscow, showed that forty-seven per cent of a sample of sector general physicians had served in that capacity for up to five years and a further twenty-nine per cent for between six and ten years.[18] These figures imply that many doctors will not have been in post long enough to acquire that detailed knowledge of the socio-economic features of their district and acquaintance with family circumstances to which Soviet theory gives a prominent place. And they lend a certain poignancy to brief autobiographical sketches given by those who did not make a move. One example is provided by a woman doctor who wrote:

> For more than twenty years I have worked in one and the same sector in the Moskvoretsk district [of Moscow]; I know every block of flats there and many families stretching over two or three generations. It makes me glad to be conscious of my usefulness to ordinary decent people and to see day by day that one's efforts really bear fruit.[19]

There is no doubt that all adults resident in a given sector are allocated to a specific general physician—with minimal opportunities to change to another. But whether they are regarded by other specialists as patients of the sector doctor and whether he is kept fully informed about them is highly questionable. Relevant to this issue is the following view expressed in *Meditsinskaya Gazeta*:

> It is no secret that unwise use of the principle of specialization frequently results in the patient traipsing from one specialist to another, each one of whom prescribes different courses of treatment, some of which conflict.
> Here the question arises: who should summarize and generalize the findings received from different specialists? In my opinion, the sector general physician.[20]

The fact that the question needed to be asked at all fairly obviously implies that the sector doctor has very limited responsibility for the oversight and coordination of the out-patient care received by his patients.

Here it is appropriate to mention a system which was evolved to link the work of specialists more closely with that of the sector general physician, paediatrician and obstetrician–gynaecologist. Pioneered in Leningrad, this became known as the sector-brigade system and gained ground from 1958 onwards. It entailed requiring specialists in surgery, ENT, ophthalmology and neuropathology to work with the sector doctor in a recognizable team. One author comments that this arrangement is only feasible in large polyclinics with a sizeable staff. But equally pertinent is the comment that it makes possible 'the elimination of undefined responsibility for the patient's treatment'.[21]

Compounding the sector doctor's lack of authority *vis-à-vis* specialist colleagues is a consciousness of being restricted to a somewhat inferior clinical function. Not long ago one doctor lamented that ... our function has come down to that of trained dispatchers—establishing an initial diagnosis and directing patients to a narrow specialist'.[22] In this situation, lack of job satisfaction, leading to high turn-over rates, is not to be wondered at.

It is interesting that some health service administrators have favoured taking the concept of specialization to its logical conclusion by abolishing the sector and its doctor altogether. But apparently the mainstream of current thinking perceives increasing specialization as affording the *raison d'être* for some form of generalist who will act as a counterbalance to the excesses of specialized medical care. An impression of the importance attached to a holistic approach is given by the following quotation:

> The sector doctor must bring together and evaluate the combined findings of the specialists. He alone can have comprehensive information, knowing better than others the anamnesis of the illness and the patient's life history, his occupational path, style of living, psychogenetic factors and so on.[23]

If such indeed is the ideal, the Soviet planners could do worse than devote serious attention to the organization of general medical practice in the United Kingdom.

So far, however, there is no evidence that the Health Ministry intends to instigate any fundamental change in the position of sector doctors *vis-à-vis* other out-patient specialists. At present it appears that emphasis is being placed on issues of second-order importance such as post-diploma training to improve clinical skills and on supply of the prerequisites for more effective performance. Incidentally, there can be little doubt that much remains to be done to equip a general physician for home visits; as late as 1969 a letter to *Pravda* complained about the lack of portable equipment, sets of drugs, syringes and so on. It also made the incisive comment that 'The state devotes enormous assets to the construction of curative institutions but in many places up till now continues to forget such "trifles" as transport for sector doctors'.[24]

It seems not unfair to conclude that the Soviet health planners are confronted with an almost insoluble problem. They recognize the value of a single doctor who has continuing responsibility for a family and as it were interprets the system to his patients. But the only personnel available to act in such a capacity have been trained as specialists since conventional wisdom denies the adequacy, in contemporary conditions, of a single form of medical education. Given the present organization of the Soviet out-patient service, a sector doctor is most unlikely to become more than the mere shadow of a family doctor.

CHAPTER 7

Hospital Provision

One of the more striking characteristics of Soviet clinicians is their propensity to admit patients to hospital rather than opting for treatment in the polyclinic or in the home. While this tendency reflects the interplay of various factors, there is no doubt that it must be explained in part by reference to the long-standing priority which hospitals have had over out-patient facilities. Evidence of that priority is provided by the fact that the number of hospital beds was the only health service statistic to appear in a comparatively recent list of forty-four indicators of the Soviet Union's socio-economic development.[1]

CONTINUING EXPANSION

Before the Second World War, the building of in-patient accommodation (and out-patient units) had been taking place on a truly massive scale as part of the 'great leap forward' in which industrialization and urbanization proceeded at a forced and rapid pace. During the war, as is still frequently emphasized, the German invasion and occupation of Soviet territory brought about crippling losses of capital equipment of all kinds, including health service institutions. By 1950, nonetheless, the bed-to-population ratio was higher than ten years before and stood at 55.7 per 10,000 persons, which was roughly half the level obtaining in Britain.

Throughout the subsequent decades vast additions were made to the total bed complement and, as can be seen from Table 7.1, the ratio of beds to population had more than doubled by 1974, to stand at 115.8 per 10,000 persons. So within a comparatively short period of time, the Soviet Union had succeeded in drawing level with—or overtaking—most other industrialized nations with the notable exception of Norway and Sweden. (See Appendix 5 for figures from selected countries.) It should be added that after 1960 the total number of hospitals has contracted, thus strengthening the pre-existing trend towards larger units.

Further annual increases are envisaged for the current five-year plan; the target for 1980 is approximately 3.3 million beds, which represents 123 per 10,000 population. Those figures, incidentally, exclude the network of sanatoria in which the level of provision is

TABLE 7.1 *Number of hospital beds and hospitals, 1950–1974*

| | End of years | | | |
	1950	1960	1970	1974
Number of hospital beds	1,010,700	1,739,200	2,663,300	2,933,300
Hospital beds per 10,000 population	55.7	80.5	109.2	115.8
Number of hospitals	18,253	26,668	26,234	24,627

Note: Beds in hospitals for the armed forces are explicitly excluded from the figures for 1950 and 1960 and are probably excluded from the figures for 1970 and 1974.

Sources: *Narodnoe Khozyaistvo SSSR* for 1965, pp. 747–8; and for 1974, p. 731.

planned[2] to reach 19.8 sanatoria beds for every 10,000 persons by 1980. But even in that year the upward trend is most unlikely to come to a halt—judging from the ideal long-term figures which were put forward as a recommendation in 1971. These proposed an all-Union average of 135.3 hospital beds and 31.1 sanatoria beds per 10,000 total population.[3]

At this point it is appropriate to note that a sizeable proportion of additional beds have been made available in premises which were not newly constructed and in some cases not even designed as hospitals. With the passage of time, however, extra beds have opened in new, purpose-designed accommodation to an increasing extent, a development which probably reflects a reduction of priority demands in other sectors of the economy. In the urban areas (and workers' settlements) of the Russian republic in 1955 only 30.2 per cent of the additions had occurred in new units while the corresponding figure for rural areas was 13.9 per cent. By 1975, the figures had risen to 72.4 per cent in towns and 71.0 per cent in the countryside.

A further fact which it would be seriously misleading not to mention is that many thousands of beds have been simply added to the complements of existing buildings without any increase in total floor space. Thus the official statistics record that in 1955 in the RSFSR 33.3 per cent of additional urban beds and 35.3 per cent of rural beds were created by this means. But twenty years later the figures were down to 1.4 and 1.8 per cent respectively.[4] So the badly overcrowded conditions in hospital, with which Russians were long familiar, may be assumed to be rapidly disappearing. (Though not so long ago the Soviet film censors failed to cut a scene of overcrowding, perhaps on account of its very typicality.)

The achievement of large increases in the bed complement have also been assisted to a major extent by the plural system of capital works planning which was mentioned in chapter 1. Various types of non-health service agencies play their part, of course, but it is possible to identify separately only the contribution made by the numerous collective farms (*kolkhozi*). During the post-war period, they appear to have first provided in-patient accommodation in 1956 and in that year their contribution accounted for 689 of the additions to the total bed complement of the USSR. The vast majority of these beds were located in the Uzbek republic. By 1960 the figure had shot up to 11,086 but, perhaps because demand was being overtaken, a decline subsequently ensued. In 1974 the collective farms brought into commission only 3,764 of additions to the bed complement. Among the Union republics, the RSFSR came first in rank order in that year while Belorussia and Armenia had zero entries.[5]

The vast amount of new construction of all kinds which is taking place in the Soviet Union can hardly fail to impress a visitor. But the excessive length of time needed to complete half-built polyclinics and hospitals is frequently remarked on in the Soviet press and has formed a stock theme for satirical cartoons in *Meditsinskaya Gazeta*. The massive extent to which capital investment plans have been underfulfilled in the health service was indicated in 1968 by the chairman of the commission on the health service and social security. Deputy N. N. Blokhin informed the Supreme Soviet of the Union that in the period 1959–67 the sum of 155 million roubles remained unspent on the building of new hospitals. He went on to note that the fulfilment of capital investment plans had been especially unsatisfactory in the Ukrainian, Belorussian, Kazakh, Moldavian and Armenian republics.[6]

So the problem is one of major dimensions and there is ample evidence to prove that it constitutes a perennial source of concern to the health service planners. Rather than document the latter point, however, it is more useful to focus on the institutional features which give rise to the problems of coordination and control over capital works. These were spelt out very clearly in 1968 by a deputy Health Minister of the USSR when he said:

> One of the main reasons for the unsatisfactory state of affairs in the construction of health service institutions in a number of regions, territories and union republics is the insufficient attention paid to new construction projects by local Soviets of workers' deputies. They do not demand unconditional fulfilment of the intended plans from the construction organizations. Many construction projects are not fully provided with workers, building materials and machinery. As a result, the resources allocated are not fully used.[7]

In the same year, Health Minister Petrovski cited an additional reason for the delays in commissioning new projects. He said:

> In a number of cases funds are dispersed in small amounts on the construction of many small facilities, as a result of which the volume of uncompleted construction increases; the facilities are not handed over for operation on time.
> Thus, in the Kazakh republic in 1968 work on twenty-one out of 115 medical institutions under construction came to a halt but at the same time eleven new projects have been authorized for the current year. The republican teaching hospital at Alma-Ata has been under construction for nine years.[8]

Turning to a related topic, few visitors from the West are likely to be impressed by the general quality of materials and finish in even newly-completed Soviet hospitals and polyclinics. This is no mere question of aesthetics, especially so far as operating theatres are concerned, since difficulty in maintaining sterile conditions has a critical impact on the treatment of patients. But in this case too, responsibility for shortcomings resides, at least in part, with agencies outside the health service which may be resistant to 'consumer' demands. It is not difficult to read a sense of frustration into the Health Minister's statement that 'workers in the building materials and chemical industries must improve the quality of finishing tiles, floor coverings, paints, plastics and other materials'.[9]

The supply of hospital beds, like other indices of health service development referred to in earlier chapters, varies substantially between the fifteen Union republics. From Table 7.2 it can be calculated that in 1950 the range was 31.4 beds per 10,000 persons; by 1974 this gap between first and last in the rank order had increased to 39.2—a not insignificant difference. Perhaps it should be pointed out that Kazakhstan had managed to pull up into second place by 1974, while another Central Asian republic, Kirgizia, also improved its relative position quite considerably. These achievements are the more impressive on account of the high population growth rates obtaining in the two republics. Latvia, which was annexed by the Soviet Union only in 1940, has held on to its historically-determined lead.

TABLE 7.2   *Number of hospital beds by Union republic in 1950 and 1974*

Republic	End of 1950		End of 1974	
	Number	*Beds per 10,000 persons*	*Number*	*Beds per 10,000 persons*
RSFSR	609,800	59.2	1,610,700	120.4
Ukrainian SSR	194,200	52.2	564,600	115.7
Belorussian SSR	32,000	41.2	104,600	112.1
Uzbek SSR	32,400	49.7	139,500	101.9
Kazakh SSR	35,100	52.1	173,600	122.6
Georgian SSR	19,400	54.6	46,500	94.5
Azerbaidzhan SSR	17,000	57.8	53,700	95.7
Lithuanian SSR	10,800	42.1	35,500	107.8
Moldavian SSR	10,800	45.1	40,000	104.9
Latvian SSR	14,000	71.7	31,000	125.2
Kirgiz SSR	7,100	40.3	36,400	110.2
Tadzhik SSR	6,800	43.9	32,500	96.1
Armenian SSR	6,500	47.6	24,000	86.0
Turkmen SSR	7,500	61.3	24,800	99.1
Estonian SSR	7,300	66.1	15,900	111.0

Sources: *Narodnoe Khozyaistvo SSSR* for 1965. p. 748; and for 1974. p. 731.

A degree of disparity would continue to obtain, even if the long-term norm for the whole Union had been reached. This is because a uniform bed-to-population ratio cannot be a practical proposition given the staggering variety of geophysical characteristics and population densities of the fifteen republics. At present, however, it seems justifiable to say that, by Soviet standards, the people of some republics are underprivileged in respect of access to in-patient accommodation.

SIZE AND TYPE OF HOSPITALS

An important accompaniment to the growth of the total bed complement has been an increase in the average size of all main categories of unit. This point is borne out by Table 7.3, which relates to the years 1960 and 1971. Looking only at the largest units—regional, territorial and republican hospitals—it can be seen that their average size increased from 445.0 to 613.0 beds during this comparatively short period of time.

In future, the average size of major units will be considerably greater, thanks to the vigorous pursuit of a policy which emerged during the last decade. This was briefly explained and justified by the USSR Minister of Health in 1968. He said:

> It is perfectly obvious that the further specialization of medical care is a complex process, demanding certain conditions, suitable organizational forms and material outlays.
>
> The experience of the Soviet health service, and of foreign medicine, proves unarguably that the organization of large multi-profile hospitals (centres) with 600 to 1,000 or more beds makes it possible to provide better for complex up-to-date diagnostic processes, effective treatment and recovery of the patients' capacity to work.
>
> In large hospitals conditions exist for the economical and rational use of the bed complement, doctors and medical equipment.

The Minister went on to note that, during the previous five years, multi-profile hospitals of 600 or more beds had been erected in many cities and more were currently under construction.[10]

As was clear from the Minister's statement, the new policy had

TABLE 7.3   *Average size of hospitals in 1960 and 1971*

Category of hospital	Average number of beds per hospital	
	1960	1971
Regional, territorial and republican hospitals	445.0	613.0
Town and urban district hospitals	114.2	166.8
Specialized hospitals	105.1	132.3
In-patient units of dispensaries (non-psychiatric)	45.9	86.1
Clinics of higher educational establishments and in-patient units of scientific research institutes	240.9	293.5
Maternity homes (excluding maternity homes of collective farms and obstetric departments of general hospitals)	66.7	115.9
Psychiatric and psychoneurological hospitals and in-patient units of psychoneurological dispensaries	369.5	448.1
Rural district-centre and numbered* hospitals	90.5	156.5
Rural sector hospitals	20.4	31.0

* This description apparently applies to the main hospital of an area which was formerly a separate rural district.

Source: Popov, *Ekonomika i planirovanie zdravookhraneniya*, p. 237.

been determined in part by economic considerations, and so it is relevant to mention an article published in the same year which gave figures for the capital costs of different sizes of hospital. On the basis of these data, there could be no denying the advantages of larger hospitals in respect of building costs and the floorspace required per bed. Thus a bed cost nineteen per cent less in a 600- than in a 400-bed unit and required 15.3 per cent fewer cubic metres. Similarly a bed cost twenty-two per cent less and required eighteen per cent fewer cubic metres in a 1,000- as against a 600-bed hospital. And the capital cost of one unit containing 1,000 beds was stated to be thirty to forty per cent less than that of two hospitals consisting of 400 and 600 beds respectively.[11] In all probability, these findings would have been fed into the policy-making process before rather than after publication.

During the course of the ninth five-year plan, the construction and commissioning of large hospitals proceeded apace. A total of seventeen, built to standard designs, were opened in a range of cities including Gorki (1,518 beds), Tbilisi (1,200), Tula (1,076), Leningrad and Kalinin (1,000 each), Alma-Ata (938) and Andizhan (750). At the time of writing, a monster size complex of about 3,000 beds—something quite exceptional—is under construction in Moscow. But it will cater only for adults and there will be a comparable unit of 1,000 beds for children.[12]

Although the concept of a multi-profile hospital is strongly established at republican, regional and lower levels, it would be quite erroneous to infer that Soviet planners have endorsed a policy of providing under one roof the whole gamut of basic specialties needed by a local population. There is no evidence to suggest that, in the foreseeable future, in-patient treatment will be provided on a significantly less disaggregated basis. The comparatively limited role played by multi-profile hospitals—as opposed to those catering only for specific population groups or disease categories—is suggested by Table 7.4, which shows the distribution of beds in the Russian republic in 1965 and 1975. Incidentally, the fact that the categories of hospital do not coincide fully with those in the previous table serves to illustrate the irritating definitional difficulties which occur rather too frequently in Soviet accounts of their health service.

It will be seen that the group which is specifically labelled 'specialized hospitals' in the table accounted for 9.8 per cent of beds in 1965 and 10.2 per cent in 1975. Psychiatric hospitals also increased their share of the bed complement from 10.0 to 10.3 per cent, while dispensaries increased theirs from 5.8 to 6.7 per cent. These gains for specialized units of various types were admittedly offset to some extent by a reduction in the share ascribed to hospitals for invalids of the Second World War and maternity homes. But on the other hand, the remaining categories listed in the table are by no means composed entirely of multi-profile hospitals for adults or for children.

It is known that the current five-year plan includes the construction of territorial, republican, regional and town hospitals of 400, 600, 1,000 beds and more. (The source does not state that they will consist entirely of multi-profile hospitals and it appears likely that they will include psychiatric, emergency care and other specialized units.) Also planned are medico-sanitary units of 300–400 beds located at industrial plants, children's multi-profile hospitals of 300–600 beds and maternity homes of 130–250 beds. In the rural areas, district-centre hospitals will be constructed with 250, 400 and 510 beds and sector hospitals of 100–150 beds.[13] From those last figures it is evident that the policy makers are determined to increase very substantially the size of standard in-patient units even at the lowest levels of the rural health service. But it is necessary to set this part of the building programme in a broader context and examine the recently evolved strategies for ensuring that the rural population has access to the type of hospital treatment they require.

TABLE 7.4   *Distribution of beds in the Russian republic in 1965 and 1975 (main health service)*

Category of hospital	Number of beds		%	
	1965	1975	1965	1975
Regional, territorial and republican hospitals	44,700	61,700	3.8	3.9
Regional children's hospitals	—	8,900	—	0.6
Town hospitals	361,200	456,000	30.7	28.9
Hospitals for invalids of the Second World War	10,000	9,900	0.8	0.6
Specialized hospitals	115,200	161,200	9.8	10.2
Hospitals of a district whose centre is in a town	142,100	257,000	12.1	16.3
Maternity homes	43,900	48,000	3.7	3.0
Clinics of higher educational establishments and in-patient units of scientific research institutes	27,700	35,200	2.4	2.2
Psychiatric hospitals	117,300	162,400	10.0	10.3
Dispensaries	68,800	105,300	5.8	6.7
Rural hospitals of all types	245,800	272,700	20.9	17.3
Other institutions	1,800	900	0.2	0.1
TOTAL	1,178,500	1,579,200	100	100

Source: *Zdravookhranenie Rossiskoi Federatsii*, 11, 1976, p. 40.

IMPROVING RURAL FACILITIES

In the last chapter it was emphasized that the average number of out-patient contacts with a doctor was significantly lower in rural areas than in towns. A comparable disparity formerly existed in hospitalization rates. Thus in 1950 in the Russian republic 8.2 persons per 100 rural population were admitted to hospital as against 14.6 per 100 urban population—a difference which represented gross disadvantage for millions of Soviet citizens. However, a striking transformation has taken place: by 1973 the rural rate stood at 22.9 and the urban rate at 21.0 per 100 population.

This levelling-up in a basic index of health care delivery was achieved only partly as a result of the vast increase in the rural bed complement. It also resulted from an increasing percentage of patients from rural areas being hospitalized in urban units; for the RSFSR[14] the figure rose from 2.0 per cent in 1950 to 9.4 per cent in 1973. This trend should also be cited as evidence of a qualitative improvement in the in-patient service for the rural population since facilities for accurate diagnosis and effective treatment are superior in the urban hospitals.

Nevertheless, the most crucial element in the strategy for improving the quality and quantity of the rural health service has been the development of district-centre hospitals. By virtue of the polyclinics attached to them they have had an important impact on out-patient services as well as in-patient care, but it is their role in the latter field that will be examined here. As a result of new building, extensions and transfer to the health service of existing buildings, an impressive increase has been achieved during the last decade in the number and average size of district-centre hospitals.

It is not easy to ascertain whether this policy has been pursued with greater vigour in the Ukraine than elsewhere but an account written a few years ago reports impressive and rapid progress in that republic. As may be recalled from Chapter 1, over forty per cent of the Ukrainian population live in the countryside and so major developments in rural health care have a significance which is far from marginal for the well-being of Ukrainians.

At the start of 1966, the number of district-centre hospitals in this republic stood at 392 and by January 1972 the figure had risen to 472. Since the total number of rural districts was 476, it can be concluded that in the latter year only four districts were still lacking a unit of this type. Over this period, the average size of these hospitals was increased from 149 beds to 212 with a further increase envisaged. It was expected that by the end of 1975 almost all districts would have a hospital with not less than 250–300 beds—or would be well on the way to achieving that objective.

Directly dependent on the size of district-centre hospitals is the number of specialized departments that can be organized in them, and it is a central objective of current policy to extend the number of medical specialists in rural areas. In the Ukraine (elsewhere perhaps, different regulations apply) the planners have decided that units with 200–250 beds should contain the following in-patient departments: general medicine, surgery, paediatrics, obstetrics, gynaecology, infectious diseases and neurology. It is intended that departments of ENT, urology and ophthalmology should be restricted to larger units. Since only eight to fifteen beds in these three special-

TABLE 7.5   *Hospitalization of rural patients in 1965 and 1975*

| | 1965 | | 1975 | |
Category of hospital	Number of patients	%	Number of patients	%
Regional hospitals	771,330	3.8	981,022	4.4
Town hospitals (including dispensaries)	3,203,681	15.9	2,158,718	9.6
Rural district hospitals of district centred on a town	4,195,665	20.7	6,510,701	29.0
Rural district hospitals of district with a centre in a rural area	3,472,441	17.1	3,825,372	17.1
Rural sector hospitals	8,239,129	40.6	7,345,106	32.8
Specialized hospitals	204,910	1.0	1,290,166	5.7
Psychiatric and psycho-neurological hospitals	182,627	0.9	308,644	1.4
TOTALS	20,269,783	100	22,419,729	100

Source: *Sovetskoe Zdravookhranenie*, 1, 1977, p. 17.

ties are required for districts with populations of 50–60,000 and since such small departments are not justified, neighbouring districts are recommended to work out schemes whereby each provides one of the three departments for the combined populations. Perhaps it should be made clear that the range of specialties represented in polyclinics will be rather wider.[15]

Although this point does not emerge from the foregoing account, two types of rural district-centre hospital can be identified—one located in an urban area and the other in a rural area. The justification for drawing this distinction appears to reside mainly in the different sizes and hence capabilities of these units. In the Soviet Union as a whole, the average bed complement in hospitals of districts centred on a town increased from 148 to 230 over the years 1965–75; hospitals of districts with centres in rural areas grew from an average of ninety-two to 144 beds. It is also important to note that the former type is becoming more significant in the total context of in-patient provision. As is shown by Table 7.5, while 20.7 per cent of rural patients were hospitalized in these units in 1965, ten years later the figure had risen to 29.0 per cent. But hospitals whose district-centre was located in a rural area accounted for 17.1 per cent of patients in both years.

Another interesting and important trend to which attention should be drawn is the decreasing role of the smallest rural units—sector hospitals. As can be seen from Table 7.5, in 1965 they treated as many as 40.6 per cent of patients from country areas but by 1975 the figure had declined to 32.8 per cent. This decline can be explained by reference to a number of interrelated and mutually reinforcing factors. The expansion of district hospitals has made available not only additional beds but a higher standard of in-patient treatment than is possible in the poorly equipped sector hospitals. Access— in the most literal sense—to the district centres has become considerably easier in recent years since development of the rural economy has led to widespread construction of hard-surface roads (the significance of which is most apparent in bad weather) and the extension of bus and telephone networks.

Large numbers of sector hospitals are economically inefficient since they fail to fulfil the annual plan for the use of their main resource— in-patient accommodation. And their staffing problems are in a reciprocal cause-and-effect relationship with their inefficiency and unpopularity with patients. Under these circumstances, it is under-standable that the health service organs should have decided on a policy of gradually closing the least viable of these small hospitals or designating them for alternative use. Some are converted into ambulatories while others have been reorganized to serve as de-partments of the nearest district-centre hospital. In this capacity they provide convalescent care or function as specialist departments, which must entail the introduction of specialist staff and appropriate equipment. Also a number have been converted for use as feldsher–midwife points.[16]

It might be supposed that once the health bureaucrats have resolved to close a sector hospital or change its use, they will see their decision implemented fairly rapidly and without resistance from local communities. But in the republic of Armenia (and probably elsewhere) such a presumption does not hold true. According to an article published in 1976, this republic, which is small, fairly densely populated and has good communications, contained as many as 106 rural sector hospitals. Out of that total, eighty-nine were so-called 'dwarf' units, with between ten and twenty-five beds. In 1974 one of these units had an annual bed-use record of twenty-eight days, another of fifty and a third of sixty days. Many contained no doctors and were capable of providing only sub-optimal care. The republican Health Ministry had 'long ago' decided to convert one fifteen-bed unit into an ambulatory, but this sensible decision encountered strenuous opposition from the locality. According to the correspondent, however, no rational case could be made out for its retention; although a Party official had asserted that the people needed this hospital, he could produce no argument in support of his claim.[17]

While the 'dwarf' units are now an embarrassing legacy of the past, unsuitable for the practice of modern scientific medicine, the concept of a sector hospital still finds a place in the blueprint for rural health care. Especially in the Central Asian republics and regions of Siberia and the Far East, distances are so great that district-centre hospitals must be supplemented by a network of sector hospitals. However, the contemporary version of these units is a very different animal from the old; as may be recalled from an earlier paragraph, sector hospitals with as many as 100-150 beds are envisaged in the current five-year plan. The construction of units of this size probably depends very largely on the readiness of state (and collective) farms to pool their resources in jointly owned premises.

Attempting to summarize this section, it can be said that a reorganization of the pyramidal pattern of hospital care for rural patients has been in progress for some years now and will continue into the future. A considerable contraction has occurred at the base of the pyramid, with a reduction in the number of first-line hospitals, while expansion has taken place at the next level—that of the district. It is true that the base remains broad; as late as 1973 there were 10,847 sector hospitals as against 2,929 district-centre hospitals and—at the apex—187 regional, territorial and republican hospitals.[18] By the next decade, however, many of the smallest units will have been closed down or converted to other uses as the trend towards specialized care in large units renders them obsolete.

TRENDS IN HOSPITAL USE

A point which has already been made, by implication, is that the Soviet health planners have attached supreme importance to increasing the number of patients who receive treatment in hospital. In 1950 some 19 million were admitted to units of the main health service and by 1974 the figure had grown to 54.2 million, which yields a strikingly high rate of 215 persons hospitalized per 1,000 population.[19] (In the same year the rate for England stood at roughly half that level.) A further increase will be facilitated by the improvement planned in the bed-to-population ratio.

In such circumstances, it might be supposed that there exists no need to ration access to in-patient care by means of that familiar device, the waiting list. But this was certainly not the case as late as 1968 when the USSR Health Minister himself admitted that 'hospitalization is not always provided in good time, especially for patients suffering from chronic diseases'.[20] In fact it is not a gross oversimplification to say that, as the supply of beds has increased, so demand has also expanded by at least an equivalent amount.

Recourse to hospitalization is to be explained to some extent by reference to wider socio-economic factors that are bound to have some impact on the decisions of practising clinicians. Thus the high rates of employment among the economically active population in general and among women more especially mean that in many instances relatives would not be at home during the day to look after a sick member of the family. In a comparable manner, the existence of cramped living quarters is likely to be taken as a contra-indication to treatment in the home and is perhaps more likely to be so taken as housing conditions have improved and accommodation in hospital has increased.

The changing pattern of morbidity should also be cited as an explanatory factor. Indeed one source states that 'The growth in average duration of life and the "ageing" of the population leads to a growth in cardiovascular diseases, degenerative and other chronic illnesses which demand prolonged treatment that in its turn increases the need for hospital beds'. Another fairly obvious trend mentioned by the same author is the introduction of complex new methods of investigation for which admittance to a hospital bed is necessary—or is regarded as such by current orthodoxy.

Perhaps greater interest attaches to certain practices or features which are rather more specific to the Soviet health service. Thus Popov mentions the extension of 'preventive hospitalization' and planned admissions of patients who are under dispensary observation.[21] He also makes a point of cardinal importance when he notes that an increase has occurred in the average duration of stay in hospital. This index stood at 12.7 days in urban units of the main health service in 1958 and had risen to 14.9 days by 1970. The corresponding figures for rural hospitals were 9.9 and 12.6 days.[22] Although more recent data collected on a comparable basis are not obtainable, it appears to be the case that the upward trend has continued. (See Appendix 6 for the latest available picture for selected specialties.)

That point acquires greater significance when it is recalled that in United Kingdom hospitals the average duration of stay has been declining gradually over a period of years. However, the contrast extends further than that since the decline, with its corresponding increase in 'throughput' of patients, has been accompanied by a reduction in the bed-to-population ratio—and in the total bed complement. Broadly speaking, this slimming-down process in the United Kingdom has been regarded by informed observers as a desirable development, tending towards the more efficient use of highly expensive resources.

In the Soviet Union too, at least since the later 1960s, serious attention has been devoted to the highly complex management problem of how to achieve more intensive use of hospital beds. Health service bureaucrats have stressed that a reduction in average duration of stay and an increase in annual average occupancy rate of a hospital bed will enable more patients to be hospitalized. The occupancy rate is the most frequently mentioned of the indices of efficiency and appears to be the only one for which a detailed time series has been published. Table 7.6 presents data relating to town hospitals in the

Russian republic in the three years 1960, 1970 and 1974. It will be seen that over these years a deterioration occurred, with beds being empty for slightly longer at the end of the period. Town hospital beds, other than those assigned to psychiatry, were occupied on average for 322 days in 1960 and for 319 days in 1974. At the risk of labouring the obvious, it must be stressed that rural occupancy rates are at a significantly lower level.

TABLE 7.6 *Number of days of bed occupancy in town hospitals of the Russian republic, 1960–1974*

Category of bed	1960	1970	1974
General	298	276	297
General medicine	335	340	340
Infectious diseases	299	311	309
Surgery	333	334	335
Neurosurgery	327	339	343
Traumatology	343	357	327
Urology	310	338	342
Stomatology	290	321	334
Oncology	306	306	311
Ante-natal and lying-in beds	290	278	274
Gynaecology	358	318	324
Tuberculosis—adults	310	301	302
Neurology	335	339	334
Ophthalmology	328	322	333
ENT	312	319	324
Dermato-venereology	322	340	338
Psychiatry	405	398	391
Other beds for adults	341	244	298
Average	332	328	328
Average excluding psychiatric beds	322	318	319

Source: *Zdravookhranenie Rossiskoi Federatsii*, 11, 1975, p. 42.

Among the practices currently favoured as a means of obtaining greater use of hospital beds is the organization of separate departments for convalescence and rehabilitation. Referring to the success of a monitored experiment along these lines, the first deputy Health Minister of the Union noted that after a ward block for convalescent care had been opened at Minsk regional hospital, the average length of a patient's stay decreased by 3.5 days in the surgical departments and by 5.3 days in the cardiovascular surgery department. 'It is perfectly obvious', he stated firmly, 'that the establishment of a department for convalescence as part of the specialized medical care for in-patients produces significant medical and economic results.'

He also mentioned a scheme operative in fifty-four large hospitals which entails extending the powers and discretion of chief doctors in relation to the use of 'labour, material and financial resources' and permits 'the application of the principles of economic stimulus to medical personnel'—which means bonus payments for the 'best' doctors and nurses. As a consequence of these innovations, a highly satisfactory result was obtained—bed turn-over increased to the extent that an additional 50,000 patients could be hospitalized. The USSR Health Ministry was summarizing the findings of this experiment and preparing to disseminate information concerning its successful features. It is only proper to add that the increase in throughput was accompanied by an improvement in the 'indices of curative-diagnostic activity' which presumably means that no deterioration occurred in the quality of care received by patients.

Whether the experiment noted above was limited solely to the organization of in-patient treatment is unclear, but there can be no doubt that the quality and range of work in out-patient units has a critical bearing on the efficient usage of hospital beds. And the deputy Health Minister reported that fuller examination of patients before hospitalization was being expanded at the first and second medical institutes in Moscow and at curative-prophylactic institutions in Moscow, Leningrad, Kiev, Kishinev and other large towns. As a result of more detailed initial investigations, the average period of treatment in hospitals 51 and 52 in Moscow had been reduced by 1.2 and 1.7 days respectively. In the polyclinics of Kiev it has become a compulsory procedure for patients to receive laboratory, x-ray, functional diagnostic and other examinations before being admitted to hospital. An improvement in coordination of services was achieved by means of the participation in pre-hospital investigations of staff from the units to which patients subsequently proceeded; this measure was said to be especially effective.[23]

Nevertheless, it seems that innovations of this kind encounter substantial difficulties if they have not been initiated from the highest organizational levels. Such is the conclusion that can be drawn from the experience of Professor N. A. Lopatkin, the head of a Moscow urological hospital. In 1973 he commenced an experiment which involved performing diagnostic tests on an out-patient as against an in-patient basis; the necessary equipment and staff were moved to a consultative clinic. During the second year of the experiment, a total of 593 people underwent a range of tests for which hospitalization would previously have been necessary. Only 213 were subsequently operated on and the others received at home courses of treatment which could normally only be provided in hospital. The new arrangements enabled Lopatkin's hospital to achieve a thirty per-cent increase in the throughput of patients. But despite this success, the consultative clinic had to be discontinued in November 1974 apparently on the ground that it violated certain 'outdated regulations'.[24]

Reference can finally be made to the recognition that, even without such organizational changes, improvements in the diagnostic activity of polyclinics can obviate hospitalization altogether in the case of some patients. In 1974 Health Minister Petrovski stated that, according to assessments carried out by experts in a number of regional towns, five to six per cent of patients admitted to hospital had no need to be there. A related point concerns the competence of polyclinic clinicians; their diagnoses were not confirmed in thirteen to eighteen per cent of cases admitted to hospital. Moreover, among those seen in the polyclinic before hospitalization only fifty-seven per cent had been fully investigated.[25]

Fully consistent with the statistics given above, and with the high hospitalization rate, is the fact that only some eighty per cent of all episodes of illness are treated from start to finish in the community. This figure, which is well below the equivalent one for Britain, brings the discussion back once more to the effects of specialization in Soviet medical practice. For out-patient specialists can hardly avoid a presumption that more sophisticated and effective treatment is available in hospital and as a consequence are all the more prepared to relinquish clinical responsibility to colleagues working at a higher level of medical technology. The absence of a countervailing force in the form of generalist doctors practising from an independent institutional base surely constitutes another and substantial reason why the Soviet health service has become hospital-centred to a remarkable extent.

CHAPTER 8

Functions of the Service

The starting point for this chapter is the typology of social welfare systems outlined by Professor Richard Titmuss in the posthumously edited text of his introductory lectures on social policy. There he identifies the residual welfare model, the institutional redistributive model and the industrial achievement–performance model. The last-mentioned is described in the following words:

> This incorporates a significant role for social welfare institutions as adjuncts of the economy. It holds that social needs should be met on the basis of merit, work performance and productivity. It is derived from various economic and psychological theories concerned with incentives, effort and reward, and the formation of class and group loyalties.[1]

Titmuss does not state explicitly that there is one contemporary state which provides an example *par excellence* of the industrial achievement–performance model. But such a view might be imputed on the basis of his statement that 'Soviet Russia ... has fashioned a model of social welfare which is based, in large measure, on the principles of work–performance, achievement and meritocratic selection'.[2] It is the purpose of this chapter to enquire how far those principles can be said to apply specifically in respect of the organization and delivery of Soviet medical care.

SEGREGATED SERVICES

Reference can first be made to a sub-system of the main health
110

service which has not been examined so far in this study. The sub-system in question consists of hospitals, polyclinics, sanatoria and so on that are intended solely for the use of members of the Party and government elite. Although the facilities are not mentioned by the authors of textbooks, their unobtrusive existence is very much an open secret in the Soviet Union.

The best-known of them is the Moscow *Kremlinovka*, a name which even appears from time to time in the Western press. Other units are located in the larger towns of the Soviet Union, and in secluded rural or coastal settings. It is understandable that there should be a special division of the USSR Health Ministry—it is known as 'the Fourth'—responsible for exercising direct control over this network.

On *a priori* grounds one could conclude that the Soviet *nachalstvo* (administrative and political elite) enjoy better-quality medical care in these separate facilities than does the average citizen in ordinary health service institutions. Empirical data bears out this conclusion, albeit with an interesting complication. Thus it is clear that doctors employed in the Fourth Department units are selected partly for their record of political reliability—and this may not correlate at all highly with professional competence. Nonetheless, as Robert Kaiser points out, deficiencies in the qualifications and skills of such staff are overcome by calling in leading specialists on a consultancy basis. Kaiser quotes a Soviet surgeon as saying: 'All the professors at our medical institute were used as consultants to the Fourth Department ... The *nachalstvo* know that in a difficult situation they'll get a good doctor'.[3]

On the basis of what has been said above, it is evident that segregated services afford a substantial degree of advantage to a limited number of persons by virtue of their achieved status. Now it might be argued that no high-income nation has a single monolithic health service to which all citizens have complete equality of access. In the United Kingdom, certainly, patients who have no wish to be treated free of charge under the National Health Service can pay the doctor of their choice privately for treatment in the community or in hospital. But the advantages of doing so are widely regarded as questionable and the view that, in general, a private patient does not receive superior medical care has the elements of a self-fulfilling prophesy. By contrast, the Soviet state has institutionalized for an elite high-quality provision which by its very nature is rigidly exclusive and can only serve to perpetuate, if not harden, existing socio-economic differentials.

A rather more complex picture emerges from an examination of administratively separate services for certain groups of workers. A number of schemes are probably intended quite straightforwardly as a means of supplying preferential care for staff in high-status ministries and comparable public agencies. But some can also be explained in terms of the special requirements of a given occupational group. A case in point is the extensive network of units for those who work on Soviet railways or are engaged on the massive task of constructing the new trans-Siberian railway known as the Baikal–Amur *magistral* (main line). In 1975 this network was reported to consist of 6,000 curative-prophylactic institutions with a total of 126,000 staff of whom 34,000 were doctors. The source went on to note that various organizational shortcomings, which need not be described here, results in some impairment of the quality of treatment.[4]

For all that, however, there is anecdotal evidence that certain hospitals for railway workers are considered to provide such high-quality care that workers from other sectors of the economy occasionally seek admission by back-door methods. Further evidence of the superiority of separate services is provided by a contribution to the public discussion which took place in 1969 on the draft law relating to the health service. The Health Minister of the Belorussian republic wrote:

> It seems to me that we have had an excessive proliferation of small departmental medical services both within the system of the Ministry of Health and outside it. In Belorussia, for example, the waterways are very restricted, yet in several towns a service for water-transport workers which consists of a single trifling poly-clinic managed to get established. The splintering into all kinds of departmental services slows down the development of specialized care and prevents sensible concentration of cadres and manoeuvr-ing of manpower resources. Article 10 of the draft [article 9 in the final version] opens up certain loopholes for the continued departmental splintering of health service institutions. One cannot agree with this. Our medicine today is at a sufficiently high level to provide skilled care to all the people, irrespective of the sphere of the national economy in which they work.[5]

It is clear that the Minister, Dr N. Savchenko, was advancing a twofold criticism; he objected to the splintering of services on account of the technocratic planning problems which this engendered, but he was also making a value-judgment—and a most significant one. Implicitly, at any rate, he condemned institutional arrangements which permit better-quality care to be obtained by specific socio-occupational groups. It is unlikely that official publications contain any comparably authoritative attacks on inequality in the delivery of medical care.

In stark contrast to the provisions discussed so far is the low-quality medical care received by those inmates of Soviet penal institutions whose 'crime' consists in being peaceful opponents of the political and intellectual orthodoxy. To list individual instances of neglect or seriously inadequate treatment of Soviet dissenters would not be appropriate in this study. Nevertheless, the point must be made that there is reliable evidence not only of inadequate medical attention but even of deliberate and systematic maltreatment by Soviet doctors.

Indeed, as Amnesty International has revealed, prisoners of conscience detained in psychiatric prison-hospitals are subject to abuses of medical science which are comparable in their inhumanity to those perpetrated by the Nazi regime. Directly relevant to the issue of maltreatment—whether by drugs or other means— is the fact that psychiatric prison-hospitals are subordinated not to the USSR Health Ministry but to the Ministry of Internal Affairs (MVD). According to Amnesty International, many of the psychiatrists working in them hold the rank of officer of the MVD and may have no formal qualification in psychiatry. The orderlies, who exercise considerable power, are frequently convicted criminals recruited from corrective labour institutions.[6]

It should be added that although criminal law procedures are used in the case of many dissidents, the civil law provides no effective check on the misuse of diagnostic labels by Soviet psychiatrists. While compulsory powers of detention may be regarded as unavoidable in any developed nation, the Soviet provisions are unduly weighted towards the authority of the state, as against the rights of the individual. The relevant section of the Russian republic's health service law (based on the 1969 legislation mentioned earlier) consists of the following statements:

Psychiatric patients are required to undergo compulsory dispensary observation and treatment.

In the case of obvious danger from actions of a psychiatric patient for persons in the vicinity or for the patient himself, the organs and institutions of the health service have the right through the procedure for emergency psychiatric treatment to place the patient in a psychiatric (psychoneurological) institution without his or her consent and without the consent of the spouse, relatives, guardian or foster parent. In this case the patient must be examined within twenty-four hours by a commission of psychiatrists which considers the question of the lawfulness of hospitalization and determines the need for the patient's continued stay in a psychiatric (psychoneurological) institution.

The organs for internal affairs are required to cooperate with the organs and institutions of the health service in respect of the hospitalization of psychiatric patients.[7]

The basic disadvantage of the arrangement described above is that it allows the patient no opportunity of appeal to an independent adjudicatory authority. (In England and Wales, appeals can be made to the mental health review tribunals whose statutory origin is the Mental Health Act, 1959.) In the absence of such an external check, the system is free to endorse the validity of its own judgments, and in certain cases this involves the abuse of psychiatric diagnosis to support the state's repressive policies.

HEALTH CARE FOR INDUSTRIAL WORKERS

The pursuit of objectives defined by the state is also a function of clinicians employed in the health care units of industrial enterprises. Interestingly enough, these are the only group of facilities which Soviet officials openly describe as providing a 'preferential' service. The term 'preferential' can be regarded as justified in this context on the ground that it recognizes the programmatic priority accorded (within the main scheme) to the health of an army of ordinary citizens who are making a direct contribution to the country's economic development. But the premium which has been placed on the fitness of the economically active population is inextricably linked to the maintenance of labour discipline.

This situation should be dated back to an historic decision of the Party's Central Committee—'Concerning Medical Care of the Workers and Peasants'—which was taken in December 1929 in connection with the policy of forced industrialization and collectivization of the rural economy. It entailed giving priority to industrial workers and collective farmers; a concrete manifestation of this strategy became the health point attached to the place of work. 'The most important objective of that period', one textbook states, 'was the reduction of illness in the workers associated with temporary loss of fitness for work.'[8]

As readers will recall, the workforce at large industrial enterprises—and some are very large indeed—can now receive a wide range of care from the complex of facilities known as medico-sanitary units. It is directly relevant to the argument being developed here that the prototypes of such a complex were established during the Second World War in factories which had a strategic importance, such as those producing armaments. The singleness of purpose required from their medico-sanitary units has been explicitly stated as follows: 'the units subordinated all their activity to the interests of fulfilling the production plans of the industrial enterprises to which they belonged'.[9]

In the post-war period, these units became an increasingly important element in the totality of health care institutions. As Table 8.1 shows, their numbers more than doubled over the period 1950–68, rising from 675 to 1,451. The average size of their in-patient accommodation, where this exists, is by no means insignificant; it increased from eight-one to 171 beds over the period in question. By 1968 the units had sizeable establishments for doctors which amounted on average to 37.5 posts, of which 34.6 were occupied. It appears that they normally have purpose-designed buildings and, as can be seen from the table, the vast majority were equipped with x-ray rooms and clinical laboratories.

Comparable data for more recent years have proved impossible to obtain, but it is worth recording that the total bed complement of these units increased from 147,000 in 1965 to 205,000 in 1974 and their average size from 153 to 207 beds. While the construction of new facilities broadly kept pace with the growth of new industrial plant, in certain areas progress was considered to be quite unsatisfactory. Writing in 1976, one of the deputy Health Ministers of the USSR cited as an example the Ukrainian city of Zaporozhe where only two units had been brought into commission during the previous ten years, despite the need for more.

TABLE 8.1   *Medico-sanitary units in industrial enterprises, 1950–1968*

	1950	1955	1968
Number of units	675	929	1,451
Average number of beds per unit containing in-patient accommodation	81	97	171
Average number of posts for doctors per unit			
established posts	21.9	26.0	37.5
occupied posts	21.1	25.3	34.6
Percentage of units having			
x-ray rooms	75.0	81.3	91.2
clinical laboratories	80.0	90.0	94.0

Source: Gomelskaya, *Ocherki razvitiya poliklinicheskoi pomoshchi v gorodakh SSSR*, p. 163.

The deputy Minister also made critical reference to the average size of in-patient units in certain sectors of the economy. Thus in gas-producing plants there were seventy-one beds on average, in food factories eighty-eight, in the electrotechnical industry 106, in the machine tool and instrument industry 127, and so on. He went on to complain that enterprises still too frequently constructed small in-patient units containing 150–200 beds. (In the interests of accuracy it should be stated that the minimum size of 400 beds recommended in 1967 had been modified in the following year to a minimum of 300–400.) Where separate enterprises located in the same town were attempting to build four or five such units, vast expenditure of capital and human resources was entailed, said the Minister, without corresponding return in the level and quality of care provided.[10]

Care for ambulant patients at their place of work is provided not only by polyclinics of medico-sanitary units but also by the health points initiated during the 1930s. (In the case of smaller productive enterprises, these will be controlled by the neighbourhood polyclinic.) At the start of the post-war period, the majority were staffed by doctors and the minority by feldshers, but this situation has now been reversed. In 1950 there were 13,290 doctors' health points, but only

5,175 in 1968, while feldsher health points increased over the same period from 8,824 to 27,799. To a degree, these trends reflect the straightforward transformation of one type of unit into another.[11]

Accompanying this change of use, the concept of the sector doctor was adapted and gradually implemented in a factory setting. In essence this involved assigning to a general physician responsibility for a specific workshop or limited number of employees. A fairly generous norm of one workshop general physician per 500–1,000 manual and white-collar workers was established for plants in the chemical, coal, oil-refining and mining industries. For other productive enterprises, the norm was fixed at one workshop doctor per 2,000 employees. The personnel in question are included in the establishment of a medico-sanitary unit where one exists, and where it does not, they are on the staff of a neighbourhood polyclinic.

A rapid expansion in the establishment of workshop general physicians was reported for the years 1960–68; they increased at an annual average rate of 15.7 per cent as against 4.7 per cent for general physicians serving the ordinary 'territorial' sectors. The figures given above suggest that a high priority attached to the development of this organizational feature, and explicit confirmation of the point is provided by a USSR Health Ministry order of July 1968. The order stipulated that, among other things, workshop sectors were to have first call on the new graduates from medical institute. In that year, it should be added, posts for general physicians in workshops were filled to the extent of ninety-five per cent whereas those for their territorial colleagues were filled to only ninety-one per cent.[12]

SICK-LEAVE CERTIFICATION

Returning to the major theme, it is important to note that the workshop doctor is expected to be active in assisting the cause of productivity by means of the influence he can exercise over morbidity and the issue of sick-leave certificates. In this context reference can be made to one of the earliest regulations—issued by the USSR Health Ministry in 1951—concerning the functions of this type of general physician. It made clear beyond doubt that one element in his job description was 'the reduction of illness with temporary loss of fitness for work among the workers of his sector'.[13]

However, the workshop doctor is by no means alone in having to play a part in the enforcement of labour discipline, and staff of the territorial units, especially polyclinics, are also expected to devote considerable attention to the whole area of activity that is known as medico-occupational expertise. The objectives which underpin the emphasis on such 'expertise' rather self-evidently include minimizing workdays lost due to illness, and the return of the patient to work at the earliest opportunity. Out-patient doctors in particular bear the brunt of weighing up the conflicting claims of the state on one hand and of patients on the other.

Some indication of the priority attached to this activity is afforded by the extent to which analysis of morbidity is undertaken locally, at least where temporary absence from work is involved. One of the indicators conventionally employed is a measure of incidence—the number of cases per 100 working population. This is reported to vary from sixty to 120 cases per 100 workers in most years. Another indicator is the number of workdays lost due to illness and this varies from 600 to 1,200 days per 100 workers per annum. In 1974 an average of 1,350 days per 100 workers were lost owing to illness and maternity leave in Soviet industry. The third key statistic is the average length of a single episode of illness involving loss of fitness for work. This is reported to vary from eight to ten days on average, depending on the sector of industry and the special characteristics of the illness.

According to the same source, a reduction has been occurring in days lost due to illness (although the trend is not quantified). The incidence of infectious diseases has declined sharply, and that also applies to rheumatic fever, industrial injuries, tuberculosis, severe gastro-intestinal diseases and diseases of the skin. But an increase has occurred in the incidence of influenza, catarrh of the upper respiratory tract, tonsillitis and cardiovascular diseases. Popov goes on to reproduce a time-series relating to the workforce of a large factory in Leningrad, to the district of Viborg and to the town of Leningrad. It is interesting that although he refers in the text to a significant reduction in morbidity at the factory, the figures which he cites present an ambiguous account. Certainly the incidence of illness declined between 1960 and 1971 from 139.0 to 119.7 per 100 workers. By contrast, the number of workdays lost increased from 1,128.8 to

1,199.6 per 100 workers over the same period. The data cited for the two geographical areas actually reveal increases in both indices.[14]

The typicality or otherwise of these data cannot be established in the absence of a comparable time-series for the Union or for individual republics. But it appears that in 1968 the USSR Health Ministry came to the conclusion that the indicators were at a higher than acceptable level for the country as a whole. Certainly that is the inference which can reasonably be drawn from the Ministry's action in issuing an order requiring the health service to conduct 'a thorough study of the causes of illness with temporary loss of fitness for work

TABLE 8.2   *Morbidity associated with temporary loss of fitness for work, 1960–1971 (per 100 workers)*

	The Karl Marx factory		Viborg district		Town of Leningrad	
	Number of cases	Days lost	Number of cases	Days lost	Number of cases	Days lost
1960	139.0	1,128.8				
1961	139.6	1,194.8				
1962	126.3	1,116.1				
1963	102.1	882.0				
1964	81.4	774.2	111.7	993.8	113.8	1,021.9
1965	108.7	1,098.8	137.8	1,202.4	134.9	1,200.5
1966	96.5	957.8	129.0	1,188.0	124.8	1,137.2
1967	99.0	942.2	122.7	1,053.2	122.5	1,074.4
1968	106.5	970.5	118.0	1,009.2	120.4	1,029.3
1969	120.3	1,074.2	130.7	1,503.8	137.1	—
1970	131.5	1,247.9	132.8	1,440.1	138.1	1,540.3
1971	119.7	1,199.6	123.2	1,496.5	123.0	1,462.9

and invalidization, together with the elaboration of measures for the prevention of illness which determine the high level of work loss associated with morbidity in leading sectors of the national economy'.[15]

Since 1968, some improvement in the indices has very probably occurred and the explanation may be sought in such factors as somewhat better working conditions, better housing and slightly higher nutritional standards, quite apart from advances in the organization and content of medical care for the working population. There is no evidence to suggest that clinicians have been given crude instructions to the effect that sick-leave certificates should be issued more sparingly. But at the same time recent literature gives considerable prominence to the detailed procedures involved in medico-occupational expertise. It is to these that we now turn.

The regulations which apply throughout the Soviet Union permit sick-leave certificates to be issued in the following situations:

(1) temporary incapacity for work;
(2) attendance on a patient who is a member of the family;
(3) quarantine;
(4) treatment in a sanatorium or health resort;
(5) the fitting of a prosthesis in a prosthetic–orthopaedic institution;
(6) temporary transfer to other work in connection with tuberculosis or an occupational disease;
(7) pregnancy and childbirth.

Possession of a sick-leave certificate enables the patient not only to stay away from work but also to draw sickness benefit from the social security system. (Keeping down the cost of sickness benefit appears to be another officially approved objective for the consulting doctor.)

Not surprisingly, the arrangements for validating a change of status from worker to patient have been rendered fairly stringent and this stringency is 'policed' through a complex system of hierarchical control. Having reached the decision that a patient is unfit for work, the out-patient doctor treating him can normally issue a certificate which is valid only for a period of three days. Following subsequent examination, the doctor may issue just one more three-day certificate on his own initiative. When a patient presents with symptoms of influenza during an epidemic, sick-leave is given for a period of five days, with an extension of one further day where necessary.

If unfitness for work continues for more than six days, further certification has to be approved by the head of department in the relevant health service unit, or by the chief doctor or a committee known as the medical consultative commission. Organized on a local basis, as a rule these commissions are composed of three persons: the deputy chief doctor specializing in expertise in fitness for work (or the chief doctor), the head of department and the doctor responsible for treatment. In arriving at a decision, they are apparently intended to refer to a detailed body of officially endorsed case lore. The general effect of recourse to this corpus of approved practice, almost certainly, is to reduce the twilight zone of uncertainty in which a patient may receive the benefit of any doubts. No patient can be issued with a sick-leave certificate after six days unless a further examination has taken place. In the case of protracted illness, examinations must be undertaken at least once every ten days.

When absence from work is occasioned by in-patient treatment, the employee is issued with a sick-leave certificate signed by both the doctor who treats him and the head of department. It covers the full period of treatment and can be extended to cover a subsequent period during which the patient remains under medical supervision at home or elsewhere. This extension may not be for longer than ten days. Perhaps it should be added that industrial workers who are hospitalized in units serving the general public, instead of in medico-sanitary units, are accorded priority of admission. One can surmise that, from the patient's viewpoint, this may be an arrangement of doubtful advantage.

As is fairly self-evident, the rules governing certification have required modification for the rural health service. Where there is only one doctor in a hospital, he has the right to issue certificates on his own initiative to cover the entire duration of an illness, unless it becomes chronic. Where necessary, the single-handed doctor will consult staff at a district-centre hospital. Feldshers working in sector hospitals without a doctor or in outlying feldsher–midwife points are permitted to issue certificates under special regulations drawn up by regional health departments. Whether the simplified procedures operating in rural areas conduce to longer-than-average sick-leave is an interesting question—but one for which no answer can be provided.

It is a point of subordinate importance that loss of fitness for work can be deemed to be only partial. That is to say, a medical-consultative commission has the power to decide that although a patient is not in a condition to perform his normal job, he is still capable of undertaking other work without detriment to his health. Apparently this power applies only in respect of tuberculosis and occupational diseases. Transfer to another job, presumably a less-demanding one, can be recommended for a period not exceeding two months. Patients who have so transferred are issued with a 'working' sick-leave certificate which lasts for a maximum of two months and enables benefit to be drawn at a level representing the difference between average earnings in the usual occupation and remuneration received in the new one. Such patients may be required to use the facilities in medico-sanitary units where workers under medical supervision receive special diets and undertake supervised relaxation and exercises.

Strictly speaking, Soviet legislation does not impose a limit on the period of sick leave which a patient may be permitted. However, another procedure comes into operation after not more than four months of uninterrupted absence from work (ten months in the case of tuberculosis) or five months with breaks over the previous twelve months where one and the same illness or injury is involved. If such time has elapsed, the patient must be referred for examination by one of the general or specialized medico-occupational expertise commissions. The normal type at district and town level consists of a general physician, a surgeon and a neuropathologist, all of whom are experienced in this field of work, together with the chairman of the social security department and trade union organization. There are also specialized commissions, for example in psychiatry; presumably in recognition of the greater difficulty of their cases, they are expected to examine ten patients during a working day (of $5\frac{1}{2}$ hours) whereas the general commissions see fifteen.

These commissions are all permanent bodies and exist primarily in order to determine whether a patient previously capable of work should be formally classified as an invalid. That is a status which will not be confirmed where further treatment and leave from work is expected to result in the reestablishment of fitness within approximately twelve months. It is unnecessary to list the detailed criteria according to which patients are assigned to one of the three categories of invalidity. However, reference should be made to the fact that a commission may decide that loss of fitness for work is only partial and not full. Even some of those placed in category I, which consists of the most seriously handicapped, may be considered capable of undertaking work in special conditions, for example at home or in sheltered workshops. Regular reviews of an invalid's classification take place— once per year for those in categories II and III and every two years for those in category I.

Some of the points made in foregoing paragraphs[16] are summarized in Table 8.3. It also serves to emphasize the system of hierarchical checks and controls whose existence so clearly reflects the state's concern to ensure that its own requirements feature in the

TABLE 8.3 *Scheme of expertise in temporary loss of fitness for work*

Consulting doctor	Validates temporary loss of work capacity and issues a certificate of incapacity for work for a period of up to six days (up to three days at any one time). Refers the patient for consultation to resolve questions about further treatment with a necessary extension of the sick-leave certificate and about direction to the medico-occupational expert commission (VTEK).
Head of department	Is responsible for the organization and quality of expertise in the department. Provides advice for the consulting doctors on questions of diagnosis, treatment and the work situation of patients; sanctions the extension of the certificate of incapacity for work beyond six days and undertakes selective checks on initial certificates of incapacity for work.
Deputy chief doctor specializing in expertise in fitness for work	Organizes and controls the activities of consulting doctors and heads of departments in relation to questions of medico-occupational expertise; acts as chairman of the medical consultative commission (VKK).
VKK (medical consultative commission consisting of the staff listed above)	(1) Decides difficult and conflicting questions of medico-occupational expertise. (2) Sanctions the extension beyond six days of certificates of incapacity for work and undertakes systematic control over the justification and correctness of their issue. (3) Issues findings on the necessity for transfer to other work, release from work on the night shift, etc. (4) Issues additional payment certificates in the case of temporary transfer to other work of patients suffering from tuberculosis and occupational diseases. (5) Issues certificates of incapacity for work in connection with sanatorium–health-resort treatment and special treatment in another town. (6) Directs patients to the medico-occupational expert commission (VTEK).
Chief doctor	Is responsible for the organization in his hospital of expertise in fitness for work.
VTEK (medico-occupational expert commission)	Provides expertise in respect of illnesses which have continued for longer than four months. Provides expertise in respect of permanent loss of work capacity (validates the category of invalidity).

Source: Lisitsina, *Rukovodstvo k prakticheskim zanyatiyam po sotsialnoi gigiene i organizatsii zdravookhraneniya*, p. 222.

transactions which take place between doctors and the human factor of production.

Radical criticism of the arrangements for certification would constitute an indictment of the wider social system and thus cannot be expected in official publications. But not long ago an interesting suggestion for marginal improvement was made in *Literaturnaya Gazeta*, and from the response of correspondents it reflected a widely held opinion. Referring to the issue of confidentiality, V. Zaitsev noted that current procedures for processing sick-leave certificates meant that details of a patient's illness became public knowledge, to the detriment of the individual concerned. One of his recommendations was that polyclinics and hospitals should issue certificates recording the fact and duration of an illness but not its precise nature. In the subsequent correspondence, a man from Sverdlovsk revealed that owing to lack of confidentiality he had been forced to change his job after receiving treatment for nervous depression. Although he had fully recovered, his fellow-employees still regarded him as a 'mental case'.[17]

As for the influence of certification on that most sensitive element of therapeutic activity, the doctor–patient relationship, it has to be accepted that in the absence of reliable contemporary evidence no firm conclusions can be drawn. But doctors are certainly expected to be alert to detect and prevent fraudulent requests for certificates. Thus a recent textbook states that 'exposing possible cases of simulation and abuse of certificates of incapacity for work forms part of the responsibility of all medical workers and represents an important turning-point in the struggle for the reduction of illness'.[18] Such is the importance attached to this duty that the possibility of a counter-productive effect simply receives no mention in the textbooks. It is surely a commonsense inference that this ethos of deterrence, as it may be called, serves to inhibit the establishment of mutual trust and respect between an individual doctor and his patient.

We can now return to the 'fit' between Titmuss' industrial achievement–performance model of social welfare and the functions of the Soviet health service examined in this chapter. In the case of the segregated services, it can be said with no uncertainty that the model has a high explanatory value. As was shown, the quality of medical care received is correlated with achieved status for specific socio-occupational groups. The relationship holds most clearly in the case of services for the elite of Party and government on the one hand and for the political dissidents on the other. In the case of the 'preferential' provision for workers within the main scheme, however, the model requires elaboration so as to recognize the priority assigned to maximizing availability for work. The maintenance of labour discipline is a most significant function of medical care for the economically active population and in this regard Soviet doctors act collectively not only as healers but also as agents of control on behalf of the state.

CHAPTER 9

Overview

> *Between the idea*
> *And the reality*
> *Between the motion*
> *And the act*
> *Falls the Shadow*
> T. S. ELIOT

Foreigners who wish to form a general impression of the United Kingdom's health service will find no shortage of relevant material published in English. The question of whether the National Health Service has been 'sold short' by certain critiques—or misrepresentations—of its organization and operation is less important in this context than that such accounts are easily obtainable. As it happens, some of the more tendentious can be encountered a second time in Soviet journals and newspapers, often being used to support the doctrinal contention that even a state-provided scheme must be fundamentally defective if it operates in other than (so-called) socialist societies.

It is just such ideological presuppositions, together with government censorship, which make Soviet criticism of Soviet health care so selective, fragmentary and at times even puzzling. Moreover, as was pointed out in the introduction to this study, even basic factual information cannot be obtained for certain areas of activity. In consequence, foreign researchers seeking to offer a balanced appraisal have to arrive at their conclusions without the advantage of impartial assessments compiled by persons who have had first-hand experience of the system.

Soviet sources do contain much that qualifies and modifies the simple picture conveyed by the glossier propagandist accounts. Thus in previous chapters it has been possible to devote detailed attention to spatial inequalities in the supply of doctors, paramedical staff and other components of the service. The authorities are certainly not open to the charge of concealing the very significant differences between urban and rural levels of provision. Nevertheless, it seems probable that this problem area is illuminated by official statistics largely because considerable improvements have already occurred, or are in the process of occurring. Figures which show that rural hospitalization rates have increased rapidly and have even overtaken those for the urban population may be interpreted as reflecting very favourably on the commitment of the state to equalizing access to in-patient treatment. The same sort of consideration applies to data on out-patient contacts with doctors, which reveal that, although rural areas remain underprivileged, the trend is moving fairly strongly in the right direction.

This study has also drawn on criticisms voiced by health bureau-crats in policy statements aimed at remedying dysfunctional tenden-cies in the service. One example taken from the field of capital works is the attempt to prevent industrial enterprises from constructing small medico-sanitary units. As for policies affecting personnel, an example is provided by the statement of the USSR Health Minister in 1971 that doctors trained in environmental health should not be employed in clinical practice. Revealing as such strictures often are, however, they tend to occur in what may be described as reports of progress on all main fronts.

Somewhat different in style and content are the articles on health service questions published by mass-circulation newspapers and journals. As readers will have had an opportunity to note, a number of these articles display sensitivity to the felt needs of patients, and condemnation of corruption, mismanagement and incompetence. It is still difficult to avoid drawing the conclusion that, in general, the shortcomings referred to are regarded as unfortunate aberrations in a basically laudable scheme. This conclusion is supported by the tendency of Soviet journalists to present material in a narrow, often purely local, frame of reference. Thus the article exposing bribery in the emergency care hospital in Odessa (see Chapter 2) made no attempt to enquire whether the state of affairs there also obtained in other hospitals of the town or the region. That observation leads on naturally to the point that the boundaries of journalistic enquiry are circumscribed both by convention and deliberate censorship. It is hardly necessary to make the point that no Soviet newspaper could print anything comparable to the following account, by Vladimir Bukovski, of the appalling lack of medical attention in the labour camp at Perm in 1974.

> There were no proper hospital facilities, no surgeon, no blood plasma. An old Latvian called Kerkis, who had been in prison for twenty-three years, was sent out to work even though he had a stomach ulcer. His ulcer perforated and he lay there for twenty-four hours without a blood transfusion before he died.[1]

The absence of intellectually untramelled assessments of the Soviet health service by Soviet citizens renders far more difficult the task of interpreting such little radical criticism as can be found. There really seems to be no feasible way of determining how widely held is the view of the Belorussian Health Minister (quoted in the last chapter) that the occupational status of a patient should have no bearing on the quality of care which he receives. The same difficulty arises in connection with a compelling defence, not quoted hitherto, of the ideal-type family doctor which Solzhenitsin advances in *Cancer Ward*. The elderly doctor Oreshchenkov reflects as follows:

> In general the family doctor is the most comforting figure in our lives—but he has been pulled up by the roots. The family doctor is a figure without whom the family cannot exist in a developed society. He understands the needs of each member of the family, just as a mother knows everyone's tastes. There is no shame in visiting the family doctor with some trivial complaint which you wouldn't take to the clinic where you have to get an appointment card and wait and where nine patients are seen per hour. And yet all neglected illnesses arise out of trivial complaints. How many adult human beings are there right now, at this minute, rushing about in mute panic not knowing where to find such a doctor, the kind of person to whom they can express deeply concealed fears, of which they may even be ashamed?[2]

With those comments in mind, it is appropriate to proceed now to attempt an answer to the central question: how effective are Soviet arrangements for the delivery of medical care? In so far as the answer is adjudged over-simple or incomplete, other researchers are presented with an opportunity to offer more detailed and definitive evaluations.

A convenient starting point is the obvious one—the impressive increases which have been recorded in quantitative indices of health service development. On this basis, it would be simple enough to conclude that the undoubted success story they recount should be interpreted as evidence that, broadly speaking, human and capital resources have been supplied at least satisfactorily during the period since 1950.

Such a view is capable of accommodating the findings that marked disparities persist between Union republics and, within them, between rural and urban areas. Moreover, it is not necessarily controverted by official statements of proposed developments which imply that existing provision is at an inadequate level by Soviet standards. Indeed, the intention to increase aggregate levels of doctors, hospital beds and so on, can be validly portrayed as evidence of a purposive concern for an improvement in the service and, ultimately, the health and welfare of citizens. Much the same could be said of plans for individual programmes within the scheme, such as the following statement which relates to the current five-year plan:

The decision has been taken to speed up development and expansion of the material–technical base of stomatological and oncological services. Self-standing stomatological polyclinics will undergo further development, and the network of dental prosthetic departments and consulting rooms will be extended. It is envisaged that 460 stomatological polyclinics will be constructed and 5,000 consulting rooms and departments opened. It is intended to develop the network of oncological dispensaries with a complement of 450 beds and guest houses of 120 places.[3]

However, it is necessary to add that some of the strategies underlying various developments are open to challenge on the ground—among others—that they have dysfunctional effects. Perhaps the most obvious example of such a strategy is the unqualified acceptance of specialization in medical practice which, it has been argued, has had a powerful and wide-ranging influence on the health service. At this juncture one is brought up against the need to qualify the overall achievement with reservations about the technical desirability or efficiency of specific elements in it.

There also remains the problem that bureaucratic rigidities, official incompetence and related constraints significantly impair the effectiveness of the service. Evidence of such a result, drawn from Soviet sources, can be found at various places in this study, and many more illustrations could have been cited. It might be argued in mitigation that allowance must be made for the sheer length of lines of communication and numbers of personnel involved, quite apart from the fact that the shortcomings in question are by no means confined to the health service. But the latter observation inevitably attracts attention to the broad socio-economic organization of the Soviet Union and the order of priorities which is revealed in it. What emerges at this point is the conflict or, at least, disjunction between the requirements of a totalitarian state and the humane ideal of providing optimum-quality health care for every citizen.

As was stated in Chapter 2, many high-income societies have devoted a growing proportion of their increasing wealth to spending on medical care, however it is organized and financed. This trend may be held to result partly from the fact that in the United Kingdom and elsewhere in the West demands for a higher level of health expenditure have been powerfully and almost continuously articulated by a wide variety of social groups. The Soviet Union's deviation from this common pattern cannot be convincingly dissociated from its rulers' ability to discount and—up to a point—eliminate the force of public opinion. But there is surely more to be said about the fact that, at least since 1958, the priority rating of the Soviet health service has been frozen. Without such action, presumably, it would have proved difficult for the Soviet state to spend at the desired level on exploring space and expanding its armed forces to a degree which is far in excess of what would be required for purposes of defence.

Taking the argument one stage further, reference must also be made to the level of importance assigned to other aspects of social and economic development which have a bearing on the character and incidence of disease in a total population. Among the most important of these are housing and nutrition. Although in both areas very considerable quantitative and qualitative improvements have taken place in the years since the Second World War, by and large, standards still compare unfavourably with those of western nations. It is therefore not altogether surprising that even now the 'terrible scourge of consumption' should absorb so substantial a proportion of health service manpower and in-patient accommodation. As late as

1974, specialists in tuberculosis represented 2.9 per cent of all Soviet doctors while their specialty accounted for 8.8 per cent of the total bed complement.

A comparably high level of provision in the field of infectious diseases must also be related to general living conditions and, more especially, to standards of sanitation and hygiene. Within the last decade a major outbreak of cholera has occurred and, as many visitors to the USSR can confirm, gastro-intestinal infections continue to be prevalent. It is only proper to add that, according to the published statistics, the incidence of such serious diseases as diphtheria and poliomyelitis has been brought down to very low levels— an achievement which was made possible by programmes of mass vaccination. Nevertheless, in 1974 the Soviet Union devoted 7.7 per cent of all hospital beds to the treatment of infectious diseases whereas the National Health Service in England needed only 0.7 per cent of its beds for this specialty.

Further evidence of relatively unfavourable living conditions is evinced by a key index of mortality—the deaths of infants under one year of age. It is true that gratifying improvement has occurred since 1950 when 80.7 children under one year died for every 1,000 born alive; by 1974 the rate had declined sharply to stand at 27.9 per 1,000. In Great Britain, however, the infant mortality rate, which had been 33.7 in 1949, reached the low level of 16.6 per 1,000 live births in 1974. Whether the Soviet infant mortality data would reveal an increase or a decrease in disparity between urban and rural areas, let alone socio-occupational groupings, must remain a matter for conjecture since no detailed breakdown of the figures has been published as a time-series.

A state-controlled area of activity which has a very direct relation to the prevention and treatment of illness is the pharmaceutical industry. As was stated in Chapter 2, production and distribution are regarded as seriously deficient by contemporary Soviet standards. For example, in 1970 *Izvestiya* reported on an investigation which found that:

A significant proportion of pharmacies are unable to offer for sale essential and common medicines such as potassium permanganate, tincture of iodine, analgin, pyramidon and other things. Many in-patient facilities of curative institutions do not receive the medicines they need on time. As a result of this, numerous complaints have been received from organizations and individual citizens.[4]

Two years later, the same newspaper publicized a comparable report which highlighted inefficiencies in the introduction of new medicines. Among other things, it noted that 'Such necessary drugs as sulfapyridazine (for the treatment of trachoma), calcium pantothenate (for the treatment of polyneuritis) and plantaglucide granules (for the treatment of gastritis and stomach ulcers), which were approved for use in 1964, were not put into industrial production until 1968'.[5] Although a great deal more might be said on this subject, the basic point does not need further elaboration: backwardness in pharmaceutical production inhibits the use of modern chemotherapeutic treatments in order to save lives and cure or alleviate disease.

Shortages of drugs are compounded by shortages of even basic medical supplies such as cotton wool, gauze and elastic and rubber articles. The range and supply of eyeglasses appear to be quite insufficient to ensure that the population receives a modern ophthalmic service. Given the number of Soviet citizens who can be seen walking with the aid of crutches, it is reasonable to infer that an increase is needed in the production of orthopaedic prostheses.

Within the system of health care itself, moreover, the Soviet government's priorities are open to serious question. To judge from the over-riding commitment to programmes for the current labour force—especially in urban industry—and for mothers and children, the main health service is conceived essentially as a contribution towards national efficiency and economic growth. This point emerges with particular force from the account of sickness-certification contained in the last chapter; as was demonstrated, clinicians are required to undertake a policing role with the object of keeping to a minimum the number of workdays lost through illness.

It is true that the state manifests concern (not only through the health service) for the aged, mentally ill, mentally handicapped and other population groups whose economic usefulness is low or negligible. But the programmes for them appear to be 'Cinderella services' to a far greater extent than is the case in advanced Western nations. One source reports that out-patient contacts with a doctor by persons over sixty years of age constitute twenty to twenty-five per cent of all contacts and that, during the last fifteen years, geriatric consulting rooms have been opened in a variety of curative–prophylactic institutions. There are also units specifically oriented towards the care of old people.[6] As was noted earlier, however, the official list of specialties which was issued in 1970 does not recognize geriatrics as a specialty in its own right and the allocation of substantial resources to this field seems likely to be inhibited until such recognition is accorded.

For most patients, whatever their nationality, organizational questions may appear rather academic by comparison with the quality of the treatment they receive at a specific time for a given complaint. On this topic it is necessary not only to emphasize the unfavourable impact of shortcomings in the supply of drugs and medical articles, but also to express doubts about general standards of clinical practice in the Soviet Union. (That is not to deny the existence of high-quality work in centres of excellence.) Certainly the author has formed the impression that some curiously old-fashioned treatments—such as cupping and even the application of leeches—are still in use. Less startling are operative procedures which have become outdated in Britain rather more recently. One example relates to stage-one breast cancer in female patients where, a few days after radiotherapy, massive excisions are performed. In comparably heroic style, it appears to be normal to remove the entire prostate in male patients rather than perform transurethral resections.

On a related issue, a visitor does not require expert training to be conscious of the difficulty of maintaining sterile conditions in Soviet hospitals and polyclinics. As was pointed out in Chapter 7, the Russians themselves are dissatisfied with the nature and quality of interior finishes, but a look at some operating theatres shows how surprisingly low standards can be. When the author visited the Ukraine in 1974, at least one Soviet operating theatre contained—of all unsuitable items—a twig broom. It should be added that, while some use is made of sterile packs, the boiling-up of instruments remains a frequent sight.

Visitors to a Soviet polyclinic can hardly fail to note the heavy emphasis on various forms of physical therapy such as inhalation, heat, vibration and mud treatments. Whether these procedures have been scientifically validated seems most doubtful and they may be appropriately characterized as the paraphernalia of white magic. The crucial question of validation also arises in connection with prophylactic examinations and the dispensary observation of persons suffering from various chronic illnesses. It is impressive that the Soviet health service should deploy a vast—and increasing—amount of man-hours on these practices; in 1974 the number of people under dispensary observation was 32.5 million, which represented an increase of 2.1 million over the previous year.[7] But although Soviet bureaucrats and clinicians alike appear to be convinced that results justify the resources required, so far as the author is aware, conventional wisdom in this matter has not been subjected to fundamental appraisal.

The basic conclusion which this short study has reached can now be stated as follows. Indicators of health service development have shown a very substantial improvement since 1950, demonstrating that the Soviet state is prepared to make available to this sector of the economy a vast quantity of manpower and fixed capital. However, that record certainly does not entail a socialist commitment to the provision of optimum-quality care to each individual regardless of social and economic status, place of domicile and other considerations which are irrelevant to his or her medical needs. Indeed, the Soviet health service, inextricably interlinked as it is with the wider society, embodies and endorses a pattern of values which has been imposed by one of the most rigidly and unremittingly totalitarian of contemporary states.

Notes and References

CHAPTER 1

1   See Appendix 1 (below).
2   *Programme of the Communist Party of the Soviet Union*, Foreign Languages Publishing House, Moscow, 1961, pp. 87–8.
3   M. I. Barsukov, A. S. Dremov, A. P. Kuropatov (redkollegia), *Stanovlenie i razvitie zdravookhraneniya v pervie godi sovetskoi vlasti 1917–1924 gg.*, Meditsina, Moskva, 1966, *passim*.
4   K. V. Maistrakh, I. G. Lavrova, *Osnovi sotsialnoi gigieni i organizatsii zdravookhraneniya*, Meditsina, Moskva, 1969, p. 31.
5   The literal translation is Minister of Health Protection and his department is, strictly speaking, the Ministry of Health Protection. Here and elsewhere in the text it seemed preferable, mainly on stylistic grounds, to render *zdravookhranenie* as *health* or *the health service*.
6   Appendix 1 (below), Article 6.
7   N. Savchenko, *Meditsinskaya Gazeta*, 21 November 1969, p. 2 (*Current Digest of the Soviet Press (CDSP)*, vol. xxi, no. 50, p. 19).
8   Appendix 1 (below), Article 7.
9   *Ibid.*, Article 8.
10 It should be noted that there is one territory which does not include an autonomous region, and the presence of an autonomous region in a union republic does not always entail the existence of a territory. Autonomous regions occur in four union republics (rsfsr, Uzbek, Georgian and Azerbaidzhan ssr) but the six territories are all contained within the rsfsr.
11 N. A. Vinogradov (redaktor), *Rukovodstvo po sotsialnoi gigiene i organizatsii zdravookhraneniya*, Meditsina, Moskva, 1974, Tom 2, p. 21.
12 *Pravda*, 3 January 1970, p. 2 (*CDSP*, vol. xxii, no. 1, p. 32). It should perhaps be made clear that the Party organs recommend chosen individuals in connection with a whole range of senior posts in the state apparatus. The incident described in the text clearly represents the corollary of the power to recommend.
13 It must be inferred that chief doctors of rural district-centre hospitals are also covered by the term district health department.
14 P. I. Kalyu, *Sovremennie problemi upravleniya zdravookhraneniem* Meditsina, Moskva, 1975, p. 86; *Sovetskoe Zdravookhranenie*, 1, 1973, pp. 29–34.
15 Appendix 1 (below), Article 9.
16 Vinogradov, *Rukovodstvo po sotsialnoi gigiene i organizatsii zdravookhraneniya*, Tom 1, p. 288; *Narodnoe Khozyaistvo SSSR v 1974.*, p. 727.
17 A. F. Serenko, G. N. Sobolevski, *Zdravookhranenie Sotsialisticheskovo Obshchestva*, Meditsina, Moskva, 1975, pp. 168–9.
18 *Meditsinskaya Gazeta*, 11 April 1967, p. 1.
19 *Ibid.*, 31 March 1967, p. 1.

20 *Pravda*, 3 August 1968, p. 1 (*CDSP*, vol. xx, no. 31, p. 12).
21 *Meditsinskaya Gazeta*, 9 January 1974, p. 1.
22 *Ibid.*, 8 March 1972, p. 2.

CHAPTER 2

1   M. Kaser, *Health Care in the Soviet Union and Eastern Europe*, London, Croom Helm, 1976, p. 20.
2   Office of Health Economics, *The Cost of the NHS*, Information Sheet no. 29, July 1976, p. 2.
3   *Narodnoe Khozyaistvo SSSR v 1974g.*, pp. 756 and 758.
4   *Meditsinskaya Gazeta*, 9 January 1974, p. 1.
5   *Ibid.*, 16 April 1976, p. 1.
6   *Izvestiya*, 22 March 1975, p. 1 (*CDSP*, vol. xxvii, no. 12, p. 27).
7   *Ibid.*, 27 November 1971, p. 5 (*CDSP*, vol. xxiii, no. 49, p. 18).
8   G. A. Popov, *Ekonomika i planirovanie zdravookhraneniya*, Izdatelstvo Moskovskovo universiteta, 1976, pp. 239–41.
9   G. N. Sobolevski, V. V. Ermakov, V. V. Golovteev, *Osnovi finansirovaniya uchrezhdeni zdravookhraneniya*, Meditsina, Moskva, 1974, p. 26.
10 Popov, *op. cit.* (note 8), p. 294.
11 Article 44 of the 1969 Health Service legislation includes the statement that '... patients are sent to sanatoria or health resorts free of charge, at a reduced rate or for full payment'. It does not specify the criteria employed to determine the amount of payment due. Patients suffering from tuberculosis have been eligible for free treatment in sanatoria since 1961.
12 *Zdravookhanenie Rossiskoi Federatsii*, 7, 1970, p. 12.
13 *Programme of the Communist Party of the Soviet Union*, 1961, p. 90.
14 Appendix 1 (below), Article 5.
15 Kaser, *Health Care in the Soviet Union and Eastern Europe*, p. 64.
16 *Soviet Weekly*, 19 July 1969, p. 5. This source is quoted in G. Hyde, *The Soviet Health Service: A Historical and Comparative Study*, London, Lawrence and Wishart, 1974, p. 125.
17 Aleksandr Solzhenitsin, *Sobranie Sochineni*, Possev-Verlag, Frankfurt, 1969, Tom vtoroi, p. 461. In translating this passage I have had assistance from the English translation by N. Bethel and D. Burg (London, Bodley Head, 1969).
18 Hendrick Smith, *The Russians*, London, Times Books, 1976, p. 85.
19 Kaser, *op. cit.*, p. 66.
20 *Izvestiya*, 31 August 1976, p. 5 (*CDSP*, vol. xxviii, no. 35, pp. 24–5).

CHAPTER 3

1   Popov, *Ekonomika i planirovanie zdravookraneniya*, p. 279.
2   G. A. Popov, *Principles of Health Planning in the USSR*, World Health Organization, Public Health Papers 43, Geneva, 1971, p. 157.
3   *Sovetskoe Zdravookhranenie*, 3, 1977, p. 4.
4   *Meditsinskaya Gazeta*, 3 December 1976, p. 3.
5   G. A. Popov, *Vrachebnie kadri i planirovanie ikh podgotovki*, Medgiz, Moskva, 1963, pp. 74–7.

6   Popov, *Ekonomika i planirovanie zdravookhraneniya,* p. 174.
7   *Meditsinskaya Gazeta,* 9 July 1975, p. 2.
8   *Sovetskoe Zdravookhranenie,* 8, 1967, p. 4.
9   *Meditsinskaya Gazeta,* 30 October 1964, p. 2.
10 Popov. *Principles of Health Planning in the USSR,* pp. 146–7.
11 Popov, *Ekonomika i planirovanie zdravookhraneniya,* p. 181.
12 Popov, *Vrachebnie kadri i planirovanie ikh podgotovki,* p. 179.
13 *Vestnik Statistiki,* no. 1, 1977, p. 88.
14 These are aggregate figures for women students as a proportion of all students
    receiving higher education in the fields of medicine, physical culture and sport.
    Medicine accounts for the vast majority of the students in question. Source:
    Vestnik Statistiki, no. 1, 1977, p. 89.
15 *Ibid.,* no. 1, 1968, p. 90.
16 Popov, *Principles of Health Planning in the USSR,* p. 120. These data almost
    certainly relate only to the main health service.
17 M. Sonin, *Literaturnaya Gazeta,* 16 April 1969.
18 *Meditsinskaya Gazeta,* 6 June 1975, p. 1.
19 M. G. Field, *Soviet Socialized Medicine,* Glencoe, Ill., The Free Press, 1967, p. 118.
20 *Medical Care in the USSR,* Report of the US Delegation on Health Care Services
    and Planning 16 May–3 June 1970, US Department of Health, Education and
    Welfare, p. 35.
21 *Narodnoe Khozyaistvo SSSR v 1972g.,* p. 516.
22 *Meditsinskaya Gazeta,* 20 October 1972, p. 4, and 25 October 1972, p. 4. It should
    be added that at the end of 1976, an average pay increase of 18 per cent was
    announced for some 31 million workers, including those in the health service. The
    new rates will be introduced only gradually, by geographical area, over the period
    of the current five-year plan. Source: *Meditsinskaya Gazeta,* 29 December 1976.
    p. 1.
23 *Sovetskoe Zdravookhranenie,* 12, 1970, p. 36.
24 *Ibid.,* 7, 1968, pp. 28–33.
25 *Ibid.,* 10, 1968, pp. 40–4.
26 *Ibid.,* 10, 1968, pp. 34–7.

CHAPTER 4

1   *Meditsinskaya Gazeta,* 27 June 1968, p. 2 (*CDSP,* vol. xx, no. 26, p. 17).
2   H. Muller-Dietz, *Review of Soviet Medical Sciences,* vol. 1, 1964, no. 3, p. 18.
3   *Meditsinskaya Gazeta,* 1 December 1971, p. 2.
4   *Zdravookhranenie Rossiskoi Federatsii,* 5, 1969, p. 33.
5   *Meditsinskaya Gazeta,* 21 November 1975. p. 2.
6   Solzhenitsin, *Sobranie Sochineni,* Tom vtoroi, p. 67.
7   *Meditsinskaya Gazeta,* 14 November 1969, p. 3 (*CDSP,* vol. xxi, no. 50, p. 17).
8   G. A. Popov, *Problemi vrachebnikh kadrov,* Meditsina, Moskva, 1974, pp. 51–6.
9   *Sovetskoe Zdravookhranenie,* 5, 1969, p. 18.
10 *Zdravookhranenie Rossiskoi Federatsii,* 5, 1969, p. 34.
11 *Meditsinskaya Gazeta,* 27 June 1968, p. 3 (*CDSP,* vol. xx, no. 26, p. 20).
12 *Zdravookhranenie Rossiskoi Federatsii,* 5, 1969, pp. 34–5.
13 *Meditsinskaya Gazeta,* 1 September 1976, p. 1.
14 *Sovetskoe Zdravookhranenie,* 2, 1972, p. 6.

15   *Zdravookhranenie Rossiskoi Federatsii*, 1, 1977, pp. 41–5. It should be added that by 1974 health care institutions were debarred from transferring newly qualified staff undertaking compulsory service to work not connected with their specialty, unless permission had been obtained from the appropriate ministry or department. If this regulation had been in force for some years before 1974, the evidence quoted in the text indicates that it was sometimes contravened. Source: *Meditsinskaya Gazeta*, 15 February 1974, p. 4.
16   *Meditsinskaya Gazeta*, 24 September 1976, p. 1.
17   *Sovetskoe Zdravookhranenie*, 1, 1976, p. 7.
18   As note 11.
19   Vinogradov, *Rukovodstvo po sotsialnoi gigiene i organizatsii zdravookhraneniya*, Tom 2, p. 30.
20   *Meditsinskaya Gazeta*, 1 December 1976, p. 3.
21   E. M. Barkman, Ya. I. Rodov, *Upravlenie Bolnitsei*, Meditsina, Moskva, 1972, pp. 212–18.
22   V. V. Golovteev, P. I. Kalyu, I. V. Pustovoi, *Osnovi ekonomiki sovetskovo zdravookhraneniya*, Meditsina, Moskva, 1974, p. 125.

CHAPTER 5

1   Golovteev, *Osnovi ekonomiki sovetskovo zdravookhraneniya*, pp. 127–8.
2   *Sovetskaya Meditsina*, 1, 1977, p. 8.
3   *Meditsinskaya Gazeta*, 17 December 1975, p. 1.
4   *Sovetskoe Zdravookhranenie*, 1, 1976, p. 8; 3, 1977, p. 5.
5   World Health Organization, Public Health Papers 56, *The Training and Utilization of Feldshers in the USSR*, Geneva, 1974, p. 11.
6   Popov, *Problemi vrachebnikh kadrov*, p. 118, and *Ekonomika i planirovanie zdravookhraneniya*, p. 179.
7   G. L. Gomelskaya, E. Ya. Kagan, E. A. Loginova, M. S. Brodski, *Ocherki razvitiya poliklinicheskoi pomoshchi v gorodakh SSSR*, Meditsina, Moskva, 1971, p. 148.
8   *Sovetskaya Meditsina*, 3, 1976, p. 4.
9   M. G. Field, *Doctor and Patient in Soviet Russia*, Harvard University Press, 1957, pp. 50–4.
10   *Zdravookhranenie Rossiskoi Federatsii*, 10, 1970, p. 13.
11   Popov, *Vrachebnie kadri i planirovanie ikh podgotovki*, p. 86.
12   *Sovetskoe Zdravookhanenie*, 1, 1969, p. 8.
13   *Pravda*, 3 September 1975, p. 2 (*CDSP*, vol. XXVII, no. 35, p. 18).
14   *Zdravookhranenie Rossiskoi Federatsii*, 10, 1975, pp. 27–31.
15   World Health Organization, *The Training and Utilization of Feldshers in the USSR*, p. 19.
16   E. R. Agaev, V. V. Bodireva, *Selski vrachebni uchastok*, Meditsina, Moskva, 1975, pp. 28–30 and 107–12.
17   *Sovetskoe Zdravookhranenie*, 1, 1977, p. 21.
18   *Meditsinskaya Gazeta*, 22 September 1966, p. 2.
19   *Ibid.*, 4 April 1967, p. 2.
20   *Ibid.*, 22 February 1974, p. 2.

CHAPTER 6

1 Popov, *Ekonomika i planirovanie zdravookhraneniya*, pp. 152 and 158.
2 S. Ya. Freidlin, *Kurs lektsii po organizatsii zdravookhraneniya*, Medgiz, Leningrad, 1963, p. 141.
3 Gomelskaya, *Ocherki razvitiya poliklinicheskoi pomoshchi v gorodakh SSSR*, pp. 130–1.
4 *Ibid.*, pp. 135–6.
5 Freidlin, *op. cit.*, p. 142.
6 Gomelskaya, *op. cit.*, pp. 139–40.
7 *Sovetskoe Zdravookhranenie*, 6, 1971, p. 5.
8 *Ibid.*, 1, 1969, p. 7.
9 *Ibid.*, 1, 1976, p. 5.
10 *Sovetskaya Kultura*, 23 January 1976, p. 6 (*CDSP*, vol. XXVIII, no. 11, p. 4).
11 Gomelskaya, *op. cit.*, pp. 173–4.
12 Barkman, Rodov, *Upravlenie bolnitsei*, p. 152.
13 Popov, *Ekonomika i planirovanie zdravookhraneniya*, p. 156.
14 Barkman, Rodov, *op. cit.*, pp. 98–9.
15 As note 10.
16 Gomelskaya, *op. cit.*, pp. 142–3 and 147.
17 Popov, *Ekonomika i planirovanie zdravookhraneniya*, p. 154.
18 *Zdravookhranenie Rossiskoi Federatsii*, 1, 1975, pp. 23–4.
19 *Meditsinskaya Gazeta*, 11 February 1972, p. 2.
20 *Ibid.*, 19 August 1969, p. 2.
21 Gomelskaya, *op. cit.*, pp. 145–6.
22 Quoted in Yu. Gordon and N. Zaitseva in *Meditsinskaya Gazeta*, 27 February 1970, p. 2.
23 *Ibid.*, 29 August 1973, p. 2.
24 *Pravda*, 26 December 1969, p. 3 (*CDSP*, vol. XXI, no. 52, pp. 31–2).

CHAPTER 7

1 *Vestnik Statistiki*, 6, 1972, pp. 87–8.
2 *Sovetskoe Zdravookhranenie*, 6, 1976, p. 12.
3 Popov, *Ekonomika i planirovanie zdravookhraneniya*, p. 223.
4 *Zdravookhranenie Rossiskoi Federatsii*, 6, 1973, pp. 39–40; 11, 1976, p. 43.
5 *Narodnoe Khozyaistvo SSSR* for 1962, pp. 507–8; for 1974, p. 598.
6 *Meditsinskaya Gazeta*, 28 June 1968, p. 2 (*CDSP*, vol. XX, no. 27, p. 20).
7 *Izvestiya*, 12 October 1968, p. 1 (*CDSP*, vol. XX, no. 41, p. 25).
8 *Meditsinskaya Gazeta*, 27 June 1968, p. 2 (*CDSP*, vol. XX, no. 26, p. 17).
9 *Ibid.*
10 *Ibid.*
11 *Sovetskoe Zdravookhranenie*, 1, 1968, p. 10.
12 *Ibid.*, 1, 1976, p. 4; 3, 1977, p. 4.
13 *Sovetskaya Meditsina*, 1, 1977, p. 5.
14 *Zdravookhranenie Rossiskoi Federatsii*, 6, 1973, p. 36; 11, 1974, p. 41.
15 *Sovetskoe Zdravookhranenie*, 1, 1973, pp. 8–10.
16 *Ibid.*, 1, 1977, pp. 14–19.

17   *Meditsinskaya Gazeta*, 31 March 1976, p. 1.
18   Agaev, *Selski vrachebni uchastok*, p. 20.
19   Popov, *Ekonomika i planirovanie zdravookhraneniya*, pp. 161–2.
20   As note 8.
21   Popov, *op. cit.* (note 19), pp. 162–3.
22   Popov, *Problemi vrachebnikh kadrov*, pp. 110–1.
23   *Izvestiya*, 6 May 1976, p. 5 (*CDSP*, vol. xxviii, no. 18, pp. 1–2).
24   *Izvestiya*, 24 June 1975, pp. 5–6 (*CDSP*, vol. xxvii, no. 25, pp. 21–2).
25   *Literaturnaya Gazeta*, 24 April 1974, p. 12.

CHAPTER 8

1   R. M. Titmuss, *Social Policy: an Introduction*, London, Allen & Unwin, 1974, p. 31.
2   *Ibid.*, p. 17.
3   Robert G. Kaiser, *Russia: The People and the Power*, London, Secker & Warburg, 1976, p. 210.
4   *Meditsinskaya Gazeta*, 1 October 1975, p. 2.
5   *Ibid.*, 21 November 1969, p. 2 (*CDSP*. vol. xxi. no. 50, p. 19).
6   Amnesty International, *Prisoners of Conscience in the USSR: Their Treatment and Conditions*, London, 1975, esp. pp. 122–34. A more detailed study of the inhumane treatment of sane dissenters in Soviet psychiatric hospitals was published after the manuscript of the present study had been completed. See S. Bloch and P. Reddaway, *Russia's Political Hospitals: the abuse of psychiatry in the Soviet Union*, London, Gollancz, 1977.
7   *Vedomosti Verkhnovo Soveta Rossiskoi Sovetskoi Federativnoi Sotsialisticheskoi Respubliki*, 1971, no. 31 (669), p. 604.
8   Freidlin, *Kurs lektsii po organizatsii zdravookhraneniya*, p. 47.
9   *Ibid.*, p. 50.
10 *Meditsinskaya Gazeta*, 9 January 1976, p. 1.
11 Gomelskaya, *Ocherki razvitiya poliklinicheskoi pomoshchi v gorodakh SSSR*, pp. 162–3.
12 *Ibid.*, pp. 165–6.
13 *Ibid.*, pp. 166–7.
14 Popov, *Ekonomika i planirovanie zdravookhraneniya*, pp. 140–1.
15 Gomelskaya, *op. cit.*, p. 167.
16 This section draws on the following sources: (a) Yu. P. Lisitsin (redaktor), *Rukovodstvo k prakticheskim zanayatiyam po sotsialnoi gigiene i organizatsii zdravookhraneniya*, Meditsina, Moskva, 1975, pp. 216–17; (b) Agaev, *Selski vrachebni uchastok*, p. 65; (c) *Spravochnik po vrachebno-trudovoi ekspertize*, Meditsina, Moskva, 1972, pp. 6–7.
17 *Literaturnaya Gazeta*, 27 October 1976, p. 12 (*CDSP*, vol. xxviii, no. 47, p. 17).
18 Maistrakh, *Osnovi sotsialnoi gigieni i organizatsii zdravookhraneniya*, p. 158.

CHAPTER 9

1   *Sunday Times* (London), 9 January 1977, p. 34.

2 Solzhenitsin, *Sobranie Sochineni*, Tom vtoroi, p. 469. In translating this passage I
   have had help from the translation by M. Bethel and D. Burg.
3 *Sovetskoe Zdravookhranenie*, 3, 1977, p. 4.
4 *Izvestiya*, 20 August 1970, p. 3 (*CDSP*, vol. XXII, no. 33, p. 18).
5 *Izvestiya*, 8 June 1972, p. 3 (*CDSP*, vol. XXIV, no. 23, p. 31).
6 *Sovetskoe Zdravookhranenie*, 12, 1976, p. 40.
7 *Ibid.*, 11, 1975, p. 8.

APPENDIX 1

The Principles of Legislation of the USSR and Union Republics on the Health Service

Protection of the people's health is one of the most important tasks of the Soviet state.

The socialist social system ensures a continuous growth in the material well-being and culture of the people and an improvement in their working, living and recreational conditions. In the USSR there exists an extensive system of socio-economic and medical measures which contributes to a rise in the level of health protection of the population; free and skilled medical care is accessible to everyone, measures for improving health and sanitation are being expanded and mass physical culture and sport are being developed comprehensively.

Constantly developing medical science is an important basis of the Soviet health service.

The system for protecting the people's health in the USSR, which is one of socialism's greatest achievements, has made it possible to improve greatly the state of the population's health, to reduce illness, to eliminate a number of previously widespread infectious diseases, sharply to reduce general and infant mortality and considerably to increase people's expectation of life.

Soviet legislation concerning the health service is called upon actively to foster further improvement in the protection of the people's health and the strengthening of legality in this field of social relations.

PART I
GENERAL PROVISIONS

Article 1   *Goals of Soviet legislation concerning the health service.* The health service legislation of the USSR and Union republics regulates social relations in the area of health protection of the population for the purpose of ensuring the harmonious development of citizens' physical and mental powers, their health and a high level of work capacity and long years of active life; ensuring the prevention and reduction of illness, the further lowering of invalidity and the reduction of mortality; ensuring the elimination of factors and conditions which are detrimental to citizens' health.

Article 2   *Legislation of the Soviet Union and Union republics on the health service.* The legislation of the Soviet Union and Union republics on the health service consists

143

of these Principles and other related legislative acts of the Soviet Union and Union republics on the health service.

Article 3   *Protection of the health of the population is a duty of all government organs and public organizations.* The protection of the health of the population is a duty of all government organs, enterprises, institutions and organizations. The powers of organs, enterprises, institutions and organizations relating to the health protection of the population are determined by legislation of the Soviet Union and Union republics.

Trade unions, cooperative organizations, the Red Cross and Red Crescent societies and other public organizations participate in protecting the health of the population in keeping with their statutes (regulations) and in ways envisaged by legislation of the Soviet Union and Union republics.

Citizens of the USSR are obliged to take care of their own health and the health of other members of society.

Article 4   *Provision of medical care to citizens.* Citizens of the USSR are provided with free and skilled medical care which is available to all and is supplied by the state health service institutions.

Article 5   *Principles of the organization of the health service in the USSR.* Protection of the health of the population in the USSR is ensured by a system of socio-economic and medico-sanitary measures and is implemented by:
(1) undertaking extensive measures for improving health conditions and preventing illness, with special concern for protecting the health of the growing generation;
(2) the creation of suitable sanitary-hygienic conditions at work and in everyday life, eliminating causes of industrial injuries, occupational diseases and also other factors that have an injurious influence on health;
(3) undertaking measures to create a more healthy environment, to ensure the sanitary protection of expanses of water, the soil and the atmosphere;
(4) planned development of the network of health service institutions and enterprises of the medical industry;
(5) satisfaction of the population's requirements for all kinds of medical care free of charge; an increase in the quality and culture of medical care; the gradual expansion of dispenserization of the population; the development of specialized medical care;
(6) the free supply of curative and diagnostic means during in-patient treatment and the gradual extension of curative means supplied free of charge or at a reduced rate in other forms of medical care;
(7) expansion of the network of sanatoria, prophylactoria, rest homes, guest houses, tourist facilities and other establishments for the treatment and recreation of workers;
(8) physical and hygienic education of citizens; the development of mass physical culture and sport;
(9) the development of science, the planned conduct of scientific research, training of scientific cadres and highly skilled specialists in the field of health;
(10) utilization in the activity of health service institutions of the achievements of science, technology and medical practice, and the equipping of these institutions with the latest apparatus;
(11) the development of scientific–hygienic principles for the diet of the population;
(12) the extensive participation of public organizations and collectives of workers in the health protection of the population.

Article 6   *Jurisdiction of the Soviet Union in the field of the health service.* The Soviet Union, as represented by its higher organs of state power and organs of state administration in the field of the health service, has jurisdiction over:

(1) the establishment of all-Union plans for the development of the health service and for carrying out measures for improving health conditions;

(2) the establishment of all-Union plans for the development of scientific research, for devising new preparations and equipment of a medical description, for co-ordinating this research and work and for introducing into medical practice the achievements of science and new methods of diagnosis, treatment and prevention;

(3) the establishment of all-Union plans for the development of medical and pharmaceutical education, the distribution of specialists graduating from higher medical and pharmaceutical educational establishments, the training of scientific cadres, the advanced training of medical and pharmaceutical workers; the establishment of medical and pharmaceutical qualifications and the duration of training of medical and pharmaceutical workers;

(4) the establishment of all-Union plans for the production and distribution of the products of the medical industry among the Union republics and USSR ministries and departments, for the export and import of medicines, medical equipment and other items of a medical description;

(5) the provision of a uniform technical policy in the field of the medical industry and the establishment of uniform medico-technological requirements for the design of health service institutions; the confirmation of governmental and economic-sector (*otraslevikh*) standards and technical specifications for products of a medical description and confirmation of the prices for these products; the organization of control over the quality of products of a medical description manufactured in the USSR and imported from abroad; determination of the volume of production of narcotic substances and the organization of control over their circulation and use;

(6) the administration of the organs and institutions of the health service of the Soviet Union; the management of those medical-industry enterprises, higher medical and pharmaceutical educational establishments and institutes for the advanced training of doctors which are under Union jurisdiction;

(7) the confirmation of all-Union sanitary–hygienic and sanitary–antiepidemic regulations and norms; establishment of the procedure for carrying out governmental sanitary inspection; the implementation of measures for the sanitary protection of the USSR territory against the introduction of quarantinable diseases and also the implementation of all-Union measures to ensure sanitary–epidemiological well-being and radiation safety;

(8) the confirmation of norms for the supply of medical care to the population, for providing health service institutions with equipment, supplies and transport and norms for expenditure on medicines; confirmation of diet norms for persons in curative–prophylactic and other health service institutions;

(9) the confirmation of uniform nomenclature for health service institutions and standard regulations concerning them; the establishment of procedures for fixing the staffing norms of medical, pharmaceutical, engineering and technical, pedagogic and other personnel of health service institutions;

(10) the establishment of basic regulations determining the procedure for organizing and conducting expertise in fitness for work, in forensic medicine and forensic psychiatry;

(11) the establishment of a system of uniform statistical records and accounts in the health service organs and institutions;

(12) the resolution of other health service questions which, according to the USSR Constitution and these Principles, come under the jurisdiction of the Soviet Union.

Article 7   *Jurisdiction of Union republics in the field of the health service.* In the field of the health service, a Union republic, as represented by its higher organs of state power and organs of state administration, is authorized to establish republican plans for the development of the health service and the implementation of health-improving measures, to direct the health service organs and institutions of a Union republic, to adopt legislative acts in the field of the health service and also to resolve other questions concerning the administration of the health service assigned to the jurisdiction of a Union republic in accordance with the USSR Constitution and these Principles.

Article 8 *Direction of the health service in the USSR.* In accordance with the USSR Constitution, and the Union republic and autonomous republic Constitutions, the direction of health service affairs is exercised by the higher organs of state power and the organs of state administration of the Soviet Union, the Union republics and autonomous republics and also by local Soviets of workers' deputies and their executive committees.

As a rule, the USSR Ministry of Health directs the health service through the Union republic Ministries of Health and also manages those institutions, enterprises and organizations which are directly subordinated to it.

The Ministries of Health of Union republics direct the health service through the Ministries of Health of autonomous republics and the health service organs of executive committees of the respective local Soviets of workers' deputies and manage those institutions, enterprises and organizations which are directly subordinated to them.

The USSR Ministry of Health, the Ministries of Health of Union republics and autonomous republics and their organs are responsible for the condition and further development of the health service and medical science and for the quality of medical care supplied to the population.

The local Soviets of workers' deputies and their executive committees direct the health service organs and institutions which are subordinated to them, take measures to develop the network of health service institutions, to distribute them correctly, to strengthen their material–technical base and to organize medical care for the population; they coordinate and control the activity of all enterprises, institutions and organizations in the devising and implementation of measures in the field of the health service, the provision of good sanitary conditions for the population, the organization of recreation for the workers, the development of physical culture, the protection and improvement of the environment; they also exercise control over the observance of legislation on protection of the population's health.

Article 9 *Subordination of health service institutions.* Health service institutions are under the jurisdiction of the USSR Ministry of Health, the Union republic and autonomous republic Ministries of Health and the health service organs of the executive committees of the respective local Soviets of workers' deputies.

Other ministries, departments and organizations may have health service institutions under their jurisdiction only by permission of the USSR Council of Ministers and are obliged to manage them in accordance with the health service legislation of the Soviet Union and the Union republics.

The USSR Ministry of Health coordinates the activity of health service institutions which are outside its system on questions of curative–prophylactic care, sanitary–epidemiological provision for the population, the protection of the territory of the USSR against the introduction and the spread of quarantinable and ot' er infectious diseases and it also exercises control over this activity.

Article 10 *Development of the network of health service institutions, children's institutions and sports facilities.* The development of the network of health service institutions and their distribution must be carried out in accordance with the established norms for medical care for the population and taking account of the economic, geographical and other features of the country's regions.

In designing and constructing new centres of population, residential areas, enterprises and other facilities, provision must be made for the construction of the necessary health service institutions, children's pre-school and extramural institutions, schools and sports buildings and facilities.

Article 11   *The system of organization of the activity of health service institutions.* The basic regulations on the system of organization of activity of curative–prophylactic, sanitary–prophylactic and pharmaceutical institutions are established by the USSR Ministry of Health.

PART II
THE PRACTICE OF MEDICINE AND PHARMACY

Article 12   *The practice of medicine and pharmacy.* Persons who have received special training and qualifications from appropriate higher and intermediate special educational establishments of the USSR are admitted to the practice of medicine and pharmacy.

Foreign citizens or stateless persons who are permanent residents in the USSR and have received special training and qualifications in appropriate higher and intermediate educational establishments of the USSR may engage in the practice of medicine and pharmacy on USSR territory in accordance with their specialty and the qualification obtained.

Persons who have received medical or pharmaceutical training and qualifications in appropriate educational establishments of foreign states are admitted to the practice of medicine or pharmacy according to the procedure established by legislation of the Soviet Union.

Persons whom established procedure prohibits from such activity are forbidden to engage in the practice of medicine and pharmacy.

Union republic legislation establishes liability for the illegal practice of medicine.

Article 13   *The doctor's oath.* Citizens of the USSR who have graduated from higher medical educational establishments of the USSR and have received a doctor's qualification take the oath of a doctor of the Soviet Union.

The text of the oath and the procedure for taking it are determined by the Praesidium of the USSR Supreme Soviet.

Article 14   *Professional obligations, rights and privileges of medical and pharmaceutical personnel.* The basic professional obligations and rights of medical and pharmaceutical personnel and also the privileges granted to these personnel are established by legislation of the Soviet Union and by legislation of the Union republics.

Professional obligations and rights of medical, pharmaceutical and other personnel of health service institutions are determined for each specialty by the USSR Ministry of Health.

The professional rights, honour and dignity of doctors and other medical personnel are protected by law.

Article 15   *Advanced professional training of medical and pharmaceutical personnel.* The health service organs are responsible for devising and carrying out measures for the specialization and advanced training of medical and pharmaceutical personnel; these measures are implemented by means of periodic study courses at institutes for advanced training and other appropriate health service institutions.

The directors of health service institutions are obliged to establish the conditions necessary for medical and pharmaceutical personnel to work systematically for the improvement of their qualifications.

The procedure for accreditation of medical and pharmaceutical personnel is established by the USSR Ministry of Health jointly with the Central Committee of the trade union of medical workers.

Article 16   *Obligation to respect medical confidentiality*. Doctors and other medical personnel have no right to divulge information about a patient's illness, or about the intimate or family aspects of a patient's life which have become known to them in the course of their professional duties.

The directors of health service institutions are obliged to report information about a citizen's illness to health service organs when it is in the interests of the population's health to do so or to investigatory or judicial organs at their request.

Article 17   *Responsibility of medical and pharmaceutical personnel for the violation of professional obligations*. Medical and pharmaceutical personnel who have violated professional obligations are subject to disciplinary procedure as established by legislation unless these violations entail criminal liability under the law.

PART III
ENSURING THE SANITARY–EPIDEMIOLOGICAL WELL-BEING OF THE POPULATION

Article 18   *The sanitary–epidemiological well-being of the population*. The sanitary–epidemiological well-being of the USSR population is ensured by carrying out a complex of sanitary–hygienic and sanitary–epidemiological measures and by the system of state sanitary inspection.

Carrying out sanitary–hygienic and sanitary–epidemiological measures aimed at the elimination and prevention of the contamination of the environment, the improvement of health aspects of the population's working, living and recreational conditions is a duty of all state organs, enterprises, institutions and organizations, collective farms, trade unions and other public organizations.

The violation of sanitary–hygienic and sanitary–epidemiological regulations and norms entails disciplinary, administrative or criminal liability in accordance with legislation of the Soviet Union and Union republics.

Article 19   *Organs carrying out sanitary inspection*. State sanitary inspection of the implementation of sanitary–epidemiological measures and of the observance of sanitary–hygienic and sanitary–epidemiological regulations and norms by state organs, and also by all enterprises, institutions and organizations, officials and citizens, is vested in organs and institutions of the sanitary–epidemiological service of the USSR Ministry of Health and the Ministries of Health of Union republics.

The powers of the organs and institutions of the sanitary–epidemiological service in exercising state sanitary inspection are determined by legislation of the Soviet Union.

Article 20   *Sanitary requirements for planning and constructing centres of population*. Planning and constructing centres of population must provide for the creation of the most favourable conditions for the life and health of the population.

Residential areas, industrial enterprises and other facilities must be situated so as to exclude the unfavourable influence of harmful factors on the health and sanitary conditions of the life of the population.

In designing and constructing towns and settlements of an urban type, provision must be made for: water supply, sewerage, surfacing of streets, greenery, lighting, facilities for sanitary cleansing and other types of amenity.

An obligatory authorization is required from organs of the sanitary–epidemiological service when plots of land are assigned for construction, when design norms and designs for the planning or construction of centres of population are confirmed and when housing, buildings of a communal and service description, industrial or other enterprises and facilities are brought into use.

The procedure for agreeing with organs of the sanitary–epidemiological service designs for the construction and reconstruction of enterprises, buildings and facilities is determined by legislation of the Soviet Union.

Article 21   *The provision of measures to purify and render harmless industrial, communal and service effluents, waste products and refuse.* Directors of enterprises and institutions of design, construction and other organizations and also of collective farm boards are obliged, in designing, building, reconstructing and operating enterprises or communal and service facilities to provide for and carry out measures to prevent the contamination of the atmosphere, expanses of water, underground water and the soil; if the directors fail to fulfil these obligations they are held responsible under legislation of the Soviet Union and Union republics.

The opening of new or reconstructed enterprises, shops, sectors, installations or other facilities is prohibited unless provision has been made for the effective purification, rendering harmless and trapping of noxious effluents, waste products and refuse.

Organs of the sanitary–epidemiological service are authorized to prohibit or temporarily suspend the operation of existing facilities if their effluents, waste products and refuse can cause harm to people's health.

Article 22   *Sanitary requirements for the occupation of housing premises.* Sanitary requirements for the occupation of housing premises are established by the Councils of Ministers of Union republics.

No premises may be occupied unless they meet the sanitary requirements.

In cases established by legislation of the Soviet Union and Union republics and by the procedure established therein, persons suffering from acute forms of several chronic diseases may be granted additional housing space.

Article 23   *Observance of sanitary regulations in the maintenance of industrial premises, housing and other buildings and spaces.* Directors of enterprises, institutions and organizations are obliged to ensure the maintenance of production premises and workplaces in accordance with the sanitary–hygienic norms and regulations.

Enterprises, institutions and organizations must provide the conditions necessary to satisfy the sanitary and everyday living needs of their personnel.

The observance of sanitary regulations in the maintenance of housing and public buildings and spaces on which they are situated is provided for by the respective enterprises, organizations and citizens who manage, use or possess these buildings.

Executive committees of local Soviets of workers' deputies are responsible for carrying out general measures for ensuring the observance of sanitary regulations in the maintenance of housing and public buildings and the proper sanitary condition of population centres.

The militia and the organs of sanitary inspection supervise the observance of sanitary regulations in the maintenance of streets, courtyards, and other spaces of population centres.

Article 24   *The prevention and elimination of noise.* The executive committees of local

Soviets of workers' deputies, other state organs, enterprises, institutions and organizations are obliged to carry out measures to prevent and reduce the intensity of noise or eliminate noise in production premises, housing and public buildings, in courtyards, in streets and squares of towns and other population centres.

It is the duty of all citizens to observe the regulations for preventing and eliminating noise in situations of every day life.

Article 25   *Sanitary requirements in the supply of household drinking water.* The quality of water used for household drinking must meet the requirements of the state standard which has been adopted according to the established procedure recommended by the USSR Ministry of Health.

Special-regime zones of sanitary protection to ensure the proper quality of water are established for pipelines carrying household drinking water and for the sources of such water.

The procedure for determining the sanitary protection zones of pipelines and their sources is established by legislation of the Soviet Union and the sanitary regime of these zones by legislation of the Soviet Union and Union republics.

Article 26   *The approval of standards and technical specifications by health service organs.* The draft standards and technical specifications for new types of raw materials, food products, manufactured goods, new building materials, containers and packaging materials, polymer and synthetic materials and items made from them are established with the agreement of the USSR Ministry of Health and, in cases determined by the USSR Ministry of Health, with the agreement of the Ministries of Union republics. The introduction of new technological processes, types of equipment, instruments and work-tools that may have a harmful effect on health is subject to authorization by the same procedure.

Article 27   *Sanitary requirements in the production, processing, storage, transportation and sale of food products.* The production, storage and transportation of food products and technological equipment for the manufacture and subsequent culinary preparation of food products, the production of containers, packaging materials and utensils for food products and also the sale of food products are authorized when sanitary–hygienic norms and regulations are observed.

The use of new chemical substances, means and methods for the production and processing of foodstuffs, and also the application of growth stimulants to agricultural food plants and animals, the use of chemical herbicides, polymers, plastics and other chemical products are subject to the authorization of the USSR Ministry of Health.

Article 28   *Sanitary inspection of the production, use, storage and transportation of radioactive and poisonous and strong-reacting substances.* The production, use, storage, transportation and disposal of radioactive substances, sources of ionizing radiation, poisonous and strong-reacting substances are carried out under the inspection of organs and institutions of the sanitary–epidemiological service.

Article 29   *Obligatory medical examinations.* With the object of protecting the health of the population and preventing infectious and occupational diseases, personnel of enterprises of the food industry, public catering and trade, water-supply installations, curative–prophylactic and children's institutions, livestock farms and some other enterprises, institutions and organizations and also enterprises, institutions and organizations with harmful working conditions, undergo obligatory preliminary and periodic medical examinations.

The list of occupations and productive activities whose personnel are subject to compulsory medical examinations and the procedure for carrying out these examinations is established by the USSR Ministry of Health with the agreement of the Central Council of trade unions.

Article 30   *The prevention and elimination of infectious diseases.* The executive committees of local Soviets of workers' deputies, the directors of enterprises, institutions, organizations and other officials are obliged to ensure timely implementation of measures for preventing the spread of infectious diseases and also for eliminating such diseases should they arise.

When there is danger of the appearance or spread of epidemic infectious diseases, the Union republic or autonomous republic Councils of Ministers or the executive committees of local Soviets of workers' deputies may, under established procedure, introduce in the areas under their jurisdiction special conditions and regimes of work, study, movement and transportation aimed at preventing the spread of such diseases and eliminating them.

Patients suffering from infectious diseases who constitute a danger to people around them are subject to obligatory in-patient treatment and persons who have been in contact with infectious patients are subject to quarantine.

Persons carrying the bacteria of infectious diseases are subject to health measures. If these persons might be the source of the spread of infectious diseases because of special features of the productive activity in which they are engaged or of the work they perform, they are transferred temporarily to other work, and if a transfer is impossible they are temporarily removed from their work and receive social security benefit in accordance with legislation of the Soviet Union.

The lists of infectious diseases and of diseases in which people carry infectious bacteria are determined by the USSR Ministry of Health.

With the object of preventing infectious diseases citizens are given preventive inoculations.

The procedure and times for giving inoculations are determined by the USSR Ministry of Health.

Article 31   *The sanitary education of the population.* The health service organs and institutions together with scientific, cultural and educational institutions and with the active participation of the Red Cross and Red Crescent societies are called upon to propagandize scientific medical and hygienic knowledge among the population.

PART IV
CURATIVE–PROPHYLACTIC CARE FOR THE POPULATION

Article 32   *Providing citizens with curative–prophylactic care.* Citizens of the USSR are provided with specialized medical care in polyclinics, hospitals, dispensaries and other curative–prophylactic institutions, and also emergency medical care and medical care at home.

Medical care for invalids of the Second World War is also provided in special curative–prophylactic institutions, and in the case of out-patient treatment invalids receive additional privileges established by legislation of the Soviet Union.

During a period of illness with temporary loss of work capacity, citizens are released from work and paid social security benefit under the established procedure.

With the object of preventing diseases, curative–prophylactic institutions are obliged to make extensive use of preventive examinations of the population and of the dispenserization method of surveillance.

Enterprises, institutions and organizations together with health service institutions and trade union organizations are obliged to take the measures necessary for prevention of industrial injuries, occupational diseases and for restoration of fitness for work.

Foreign citizens and stateless persons permanently resident in the USSR can use medical care on the same basis as citizens of the USSR.

Medical care for foreign citizens and stateless persons temporarily resident in the USSR is provided under a procedure established by the USSR Ministry of Health.

Article 33   *Procedure for providing curative–prophylactic care to citizens.* Curative–prophylactic care is provided for citizens by the health service institutions in their place of residence and place of work.

Persons who are victims of accidents or who need urgent medical care because of a sudden attack of illness are given this care without delay by the nearest curative–prophylactic institution, irrespective of its departmental subordination.

Medical and pharmaceutical personnel are obliged to give first aid to citizens travelling in means of transport, on the street, in other public places or at home.

Where necessary, patients may be sent to appropriate curative–prophylactic institutions of other Union republics according to the procedure established by the USSR Ministry of Health or to curative–prophylactic institutions within the confines of a Union republic, according to the procedure established by the Union republic Ministry of Health.

When necessary, doctors are called upon by the appropriate health service organs to take part in commissions for the medical examination of citizens.

Article 34   *The use of methods of diagnosis and treatment and the use of remedies.* In medical practice doctors use the methods of diagnosis, prevention and treatment and the medicines authorized by the USSR Ministry of Health.

In the interests of curing a patient with the patient's consent or, in the case of patients under sixteen years of age or mental patients, with the consent of their parents, guardians or trustees, a doctor may use new methods of diagnosis, prevention and treatment or new medicines that are scientifically validated but have not yet been authorized for general use. The procedure for the use of such methods of diagnosis, prevention and treatment and of medicines is established by the USSR Ministry of Health.

Article 35   *Procedure for surgical intervention and the use of complicated methods of diagnosis.* Surgical operations are performed and complicated methods of treatment are used with the consent of the patient or, in the case of a patient under sixteen years of age or psychiatric patients, with the consent of their parents, guardians or trustees.

Emergency surgical operations are performed or complicated methods of diagnosis are used by doctors without the consent of patients or their parents, guardians or trustees only in those exceptional cases when a delay in the establishment of a diagnosis or performing the operation would endanger the patient's life and it is impossible to obtain the consent of the persons concerned.

Article 36   *Special measures of prevention and treatment.* With the object of protecting the health of the population, the health service organs are obliged to carry out special measures for the prevention and treatment of diseases which represent a danger to others (tuberculosis, psychiatric and venereological diseases, leprosy, chronic alcoholism and drug addiction) and also of quarantinable diseases.

Tuberculous patients are provided with anti-tuberculosis preparations free of charge; their treatment in sanatoria and prophylactoria is also free of charge.

The cases in which compulsory treatment and compulsory hospitalization of persons suffering from the above diseases are applied and the procedure used may be established by legislation of the Soviet Union and Union republics.

Article 37   *Assistance to medical personnel in providing curative–prophylactic aid to citizens.* For the organization of health service institutions at enterprises, institutions and organizations, the management is obliged to allocate the necessary premises and transport and also to provide assistance to doctors and other medical personnel in the performance of their professional duties.

The executive committees of local Soviets of workers' deputies, the directors of enterprises, institutions and organizations and other officials are obliged to help medical personnel in providing urgent medical care to citizens by making available transport, means of communication and other necessary assistance.

When a patient's life is in danger, a doctor or other medical personnel may use, free of charge, any form of transport available in the given situation to go to the patient or to transport the patient to the nearest curative–prophylactic institution.

PART V
PROTECTION OF MOTHERHOOD AND CHILDHOOD

Article 38   *Encouragement of motherhood. Guarantees of protection of the health of mother and child.* In the USSR motherhood is protected and encouraged by the state.

The protection of the health of mother and child is ensured by the organization of an extensive network of women's consultation centres, maternity hospitals, sanatoria and rest homes for expectant mothers and mothers with children, nurseries, kindergartens and other children's institutions; by granting maternity leave to women with the payment of social security benefit; the establishment of breaks in work for feeding babies; the payment, according to established procedure, of benefit on the birth of a child and benefit during time spent caring for a sick child; a ban on the use of female labour in occupations that are arduous and injurious to health; the transfer of expectant mothers to lighter work while still paying them their average wage; the improvement of working and living conditions and making them more healthy; state and public assistance to the family and other measures under the procedure established by legislation of the Soviet Union and Union republics.

In order to protect the health of a woman, she is granted the right to decide for herself the question of motherhood.

Article 39   *The provision of medical care to expectant mothers and new-born babies.* The health service institutions provide every woman with skilled medical observation during pregnancy, in-patient medical care at childbirth and curative–prophylactic care to the mother and new-born child.

Article 40   *The provision of medical care to children and adolescents.* Medical care for children and adolescents is provided by curative–prophylactic and health-improving institutions; children's polyclinics, dispensaries, hospital sanatoria and other health service institutions. Children are admitted to sanatoria for children without charge.

Children and adolescents are under dispensary observation.

Article 41   *Concern for the strengthening and protection of children and adolescents.* With the object of raising a healthy young generation with harmoniously developed physical and spiritual powers, state organs, enterprises, institutions and organizations, collective farms, trade unions and other public organizations provide for the development of an extensive network of children's nurseries, kindergartens, schools, boarding schools, open-air schools, young pioneer camps and other children's institutions.

Children who receive their upbringing in children's institutions and their education in schools are provided with the conditions necessary to preserve and strengthen their health and to receive education in hygiene. The work- and study-load and also the model regime of children's activities are determined in agreement with the USSR Ministry of Health.

Supervision over the protection of children's health and the implementation of health-improving measures in children's institutions and schools is carried out by health, service organs and institutions together with the national education organs and institutions and with the participation of public organizations.

Article 42   *State assistance to citizens in caring for children. Privileges granted to mothers who have sick children.* The basic expenditures on the maintenance of children in nurseries, kindergartens and other children's institutions are paid out of the state budget and also the funds of enterprises, institutions, organizations, collective farms, trade unions and other public organizations.

Children who have physical or psychological handicaps are maintained at state expense in infants' homes, children's homes and other specialized institutions for children.

If it is impossible to hospitalize a sick child or if hospital treatment is not indicated, the mother or another member of the family who is taking care of the child may be released from work and receive social security benefit under the established procedure.

During in-patient treatment of a child less than one year old and also of a gravely ill older child, if in the doctor's opinion the child needs maternal care, the mother is given the possibility of remaining with her child at the curative institution and receives social security benefit under the established procedure.

Article 43   *Supervision of work training and on-the-job training and working conditions of adolescents.* On-the-job training of adolescents is permitted in those occupations which are suited to their age, physical and mental development and state of health. Work training and on-the-job training are carried out under systematic medical supervision.

Supervision over the observance of working conditions of adolescents as established by legislation of the Soviet Union and Union republics and also over the implementation of special measures aimed at preventing illness among adolescents is exercised by the health service organs and institutions, together with the national education organs, trade unions, komsomols and other public organizations.

PART VI
SANATORIUM–HEALTH-RESORT TREATMENT. ORGANIZATION OF RECREATION, TOURISM AND PHYSICAL CULTURE

Article 44   *Sanatorium–health-resort treatment of citizens.* The indications and contra-indications for in-patient and out-patient treatment at all health resorts and sanatoria of the USSR are established by the USSR Ministry of Health.

The procedure for the medical selection and assignment of patients for sanatorium–health-resort treatment is established by the USSR Ministry of Health with the agreement of the Central Council of trade unions. In accordance with established procedure, patients are sent to sanatoria or health resorts free of charge, and at a reduced rate or for full payment.

Article 45   *Health resorts and sanitary protection zones.* Localities possessing natural curative means, mineral springs, deposits of medicinal mud, climatic and other conditions favourable to the treatment and prevention of illness may be designated as health resorts.

The designation of a locality as a health resort, the determination of the boundaries of sanitary zones and the specification of a regime are undertaken by the USSR Council of Ministers or the Union-republic Council of Ministers on the joint recommendation of the USSR Ministry of Health and the Central Council of the trade unions or of the Union-republic Ministry of Health and the republican Council of trade unions with the agreement of the local Soviet of workers' deputies on whose territory the given health resort is situated.

Article 46   *The organization and opening of sanatoria and health resorts.* The organization and opening of sanatoria and health resorts are permitted by authorization of the USSR Ministry of Health and the Central Council of trade unions with the agreement of the Union republic Council of Ministers.

The specialization (medical profile) of sanatoria and health resorts is determined by the USSR Ministry of Health and the Central Council of trade unions.

Article 47   *Coordination of the activity of sanatoria and health resorts.* The co-ordination of the activity of sanatoria and health resorts in the use of means of treatment and health resort factors and in the organization of sanatoria–health-resort regimes is exercised, irrespective of departmental subordination, by the appropriate organs for the administration of health resorts.

The USSR Ministry of Health, the Union republic and autonomous republic Ministries of Health exercise supervision over the organization of curative-prophylactic work in sanatoria and health resorts and also give them scientific-methodological and advisory assistance.

Article 48   *The use of rest homes, guest houses, tourist facilities and other recreational institutions.* Under established procedure, citizens use rest homes, guest houses, tourist facilities and other recreational institutions free of charge, at a reduced rate or for full payment.

Article 49   *The organization of physical culture, sport and tourism.* State organs, trade unions, komsomol and cooperative organizations, sports societies, enterprises, institutions and organizations must promote physical health, sports, touring and hiking among the population, the establishment and strengthening of physical culture collectives, tourist clubs and organizations and the introduction of gymnastic exercises at the place of work.

The workplans of children's pre-school and extramural institutions and the programmes of general-education schools, vocational–technical schools and specialized intermediate and higher educational institutions provide for physical education.

Citizens are provided with sporting installations, sporting equipment and tourist equipment to use for physical culture and sport under the established procedure.

Medical supervision over the state of health of citizens engaging in physical culture and sport is exercised by health service institutions.

PART VII
MEDICAL EXPERTISE

Article 50   *Performance of medical expertise on fitness for work.* Expertise on temporary unfitness for work is given by a doctor or commission of doctors in health service institutions; they grant leave for illness and injury, for pregnancy and childbirth, for care of a sick member of the family and for quarantining, for the fitting of prostheses and sanatorium–health-resort treatment; they determine the necessity for and length of the temporary transfer of an employee to another kind of work because of illness under the established procedure and they also make decisions about referral to the medico-occupational expert commission.

Expertise on prolonged or permanent loss of work capacity is given by medico-occupational expert commissions which establish the extent of loss of work capacity, the category and cause of invalidity; they determine the conditions and types of labour, work and occupations which are suitable for the invalids' state of health; they check on the suitability of the employment of invalids in accordance with the expert findings; they assist in the rehabilitation of invalids.

The findings of medico-occupational expert commissions on the conditions and nature of the labour that invalids can engage in are binding on the administrations of enterprises, institutions and organizations.

The procedure for the organization and performance of expertise on fitness for work is established by legislation of the Soviet Union and Union republics.

Article 51   *Forensic-medical and forensic-psychiatric expertise.* Forensic-medical and forensic-psychiatric expertise is given, in accordance with the legislation of the Soviet Union and Union republics by the decision of a person conducting a preliminary enquiry, an investigator, a prosecutor and also by court order.

The procedure for the organization and performance of forensic-medical and forensic-psychiatric expertise is established by the USSR Ministry of Health with the agreement of the USSR Supreme Court, the USSR Prosecutor's Office, the USSR Ministry of Internal Affairs and other departments.

PART VIII
MEDICINAL AND PROSTHETIC TREATMENT

Article 52   *Procedure for providing medicinal treatment to citizens.* Medicinal treatment for citizens is provided by state pharmaceutical institutions and also by curative–prophylactic institutions.

The procedure for providing citizens with medicinal treatment free of charge or at a reduced rate for ambulatory–polyclinic care is determined by legislation of the Soviet Union.

Pharmaceutical institutions may issue only such medicines as have been authorized for use by the USSR Ministry of Health.

Article 53   *Ensuring supervision over the production of medicines.* The production of new medicines for medical purposes is permitted by authorization of the USSR Ministry of Health after their curative or prophylactic effectiveness has been established.

The quality of medicines must meet the requirements of the USSR state pharmacopoeia or technical specifications approved under established procedure.

Supervision over the quality of medicines is exercised by the USSR Ministry of Health.

Article 54   *The provision of prosthetic assistance to citizens.* When necessary, citizens are provided with prosthetic appliances, orthopaedic and corrective devices, hearing aids, means of curative physical culture and special means of getting about.

The categories of persons entitled to the above articles and items free or at a reduced rate and also the conditions of and procedure for their provision are established by legislation of the Soviet Union and Union republics.

PART IX
INTERNATIONAL TREATIES AND AGREEMENTS

Article 55 *International treaties and agreements.* If an international treaty or international agreement to which the USSR is a party has established regulations other than those contained in the health service legislation of the Soviet Union and Union republics, then the regulations of the international treaty or international agreement are applied.

Source: *Vedomosti Verkhnovo Soveta SSSR*, 1969, no. 52 (1502), pp. 710–28. In making this translation the author has had assistance from the text of the translation published in *CDSP*, vol. XXII, no. 1, pp. 7–13.

APPENDIX 2

Capital Cities of Union Republics

Republic	City	Population at 1 January 1975 (000s)
RSFSR	Moscow	7,632
Ukrainian SSR	Kiev	1,947
Belorussian SSR	Minsk	1,147
Uzbek SSR	Tashkent	1,595
Kazakh SSR	Alma-Ata	836
Georgian SSR	Tblisi	1,006
Azerbaidzhan SSR	Baku	1,383
Lithuanian SSR	Vilnius	433
Moldavian SSR	Kishinev	452
Latvian SSR	Riga	796
Kirgiz SSR	Frunze	486
Tazhik SSR	Dushanbe	436
Armenian SSR	Erevan	899
Turkmen SSR	Ashkhabad	289
Estonian SSR	Tallin	399

Source: *Narodnoe Khozyaistvo SSSR v 1974g.*, pp. 22–30.

Doctor-to-Population Ratios in Selected Countries

Country	Year	Doctors per 10,000 population*
Australia	1973	13.9
Austria	1974	20.1
Belgium	1973	17.6
Bulgaria	1974	21.0
Czechoslovakia	1974	23.1
Denmark	1972	16.3
England and Wales	1974	13.1
Federal Republic of Germany	1974	17.9
France	1974	14.7
Israel	1973	28.7
Netherlands	1974	14.9
New Zealand	1972	11.8
Northern Ireland	1973	13.8
Norway	1974	16.5
Poland	1974	16.9
Romania	1973	12.4
Scotland	1974	16.1
Sweden	1973	15.5
Switzerland	1974	16.8
USA	1973	13.9
USSR	1974	27.5

* Excludes dentists.

Source: World Health Organization, *World Health Statistics Annual 1973–1976*, Geneva, 1976, vol. III, pp. 74–6. The figure for the USSR has been calculated from *Narodnoe Khozyaistvo SSSR v 1974g.* and is lower than the incorrect figure cited in the WHO source.

APPENDIX 4

The Soviet Doctor's Oath

The taking of an oath by all newly qualified doctors became compulsory only a few years ago, as a result of Article 13 of the 1969 health service legislation. The wording, which was determined in 1971 by the Praesidium of the USSR Supreme Soviet, differs in significant respects from the Hippocratic oath. The latter defines the relationship between doctor and patient without reference to the role of the state, whereas the Soviet variant qualifies the ideal of service to a patient by its references to 'the principles of communist morality' and 'responsibility to the people and the Soviet government'. The text runs as follows.

THE OATH OF A DOCTOR OF THE SOVIET UNION

Having received the lofty title of doctor and having taken up a doctor's occupation, I solemnly swear:

to devote all my knowledge and powers to the protection and improvement of man's health and the cure and prevention of illness; to work conscientiously in the place demanded by the interests of society;

to be prepared always to provide medical care, to treat patients with attention and solicitude; to keep medical secrets;

to improve continuously my medical knowledge and skills as a doctor; to assist through my work the development of the science and practice of medicine;

to turn for advice, if the interests of the patient demand this, to professional colleagues and never to refuse advice and assistance to them;

to preserve and develop the noble traditions of our country's medicine; in all my actions to guide myself by the principles of communist morality; to remember always a Soviet doctor's lofty calling and responsibility to the people and the Soviet government.

I swear to remain faithful to this oath throughout the whole of my life.

APPENDIX 5

Hospital Bed-to-Population Ratios in Selected Countries

Country	Year	Hospital beds per 10,000 population
Australia	1972	123.9
Austria	1973	110.5
Belgium	1974	88.9
Bulgaria	1973	82.1
Czechoslovakia	1974	101.1
Denmark	1970	96.8
England and Wales	1973	87.5
Federal Republic of Germany	1974	115.5
France	1973	102.4
Israel	1974	58.5
Netherlands	1973	101.4
New Zealand	1971	63.0
Northern Ireland	1973	116.2
Norway	1974	137.1
Poland	1974	77.5
Romania	1974	91.3
Scotland	1974	118.1
Sweden	1973	152.4
Switzerland	1971	113.9
USA	1974	67.0
USSR	1973	114.8

Source: *World Health Statistics Annual 1973–1976*, vol. III, pp. 292–6.

APPENDIX 6

Average Duration of Stay in Selected Departments in 1974

Department	Urban hospitals	Rural hospitals
General medicine	19.5	15.0
Adult surgery	13.2	12.0
Children's surgery	11.2	—
Infectious diseases—adults	13.4	14.2
Infectious diseases—children	16.2	15.1
Maternity cases excluding complications of pregnancy	9.6	9.1
Tuberculosis—adults	82.6	84.1
ENT—adults	10.9	10.1
ENT—children	10.1	—
Paediatrics	15.5	11.4

Source: I. S. Sluchanko, G. F. Tserkovni, *Statisticheskaya informatsiya v upravlenii uchrezhdeniyami zdravookhraneniya*, Meditsina, Moskva, 1976, p. 152.

Index